HEALTHCARE CAREER GUIDE

Susan Odegaard Turner, RN, PhD

July, 2013

DEDICATION

To Angela and Jordan,
You constantly teach me to think outside my box
I am so proud of who you have both become!

ACKNOWLEDGEMENTS

Patty Alley- for being a teacher, role model and sage about life.

SUSAN ODEGAARD TURNER

As founder of the consulting firm, Turner Healthcare Associates, Inc., Dr. Turner has been able to use the skills gleaned from nearly thirty seven years of experience in the healthcare field. She began her career as a Critical Care Unit and Emergency Department registered nurse. She has served in top management roles including Chief Operating Officer, Vice President, Nursing, Director of Education, Product Line Manager, and Vice President of Business Development for various hospitals throughout Southern California. She has provided transition management for organizations during re-structuring and ongoing organizational and program development for hospitals. Dr. Turner has also worked with home health agencies and long-term care facilities, joining with management teams to redesign programs for both acute and ambulatory care settings. Dr. Turner was the first appointed Chief Nurse Executive for the California Prison system (CDCR), overseeing 5000 nursing personnel in 33 prisons and 25 fire camps throughout the state.

She has designed and published the "Transitions in Healthcare" program; a step-by-step guide for healthcare providers to work with nurses for transitioning within the evolving healthcare industry, through the American Association of Critical Care Nurses. She is the author of "The Nurse's Guide to Managed Care," published by Aspen Publishers and "Nursing Career Guide," published by Jones Bartlett.

In addition to her Bachelor of Science degree in Nursing from Mount St. Mary's College, Los Angeles, Dr. Turner holds a Master's Degree in Nursing Administration from the University of California, Los Angeles, and a Master's of Business Administration from California Lutheran University. She received her Doctorate in Business Administration at Southern California University. Dr. Turner has been faculty for the UCLA Graduate School of Nursing and for University of Phoenix. She spent six years as the Healthcare Careers Expert for Monster.com and has providing her strategic planning expertise to help formulate a strategic plan for the state of California, through the California Institute for Nursing and Health Care. She is the former project associate for the California Strategic Planning Committee for Nursing. Dr. Turner lectures widely on nursing and healthcare issues. Her work can be read in national healthcare journals.

TABLE OF CONTENTS

HEALTHCARE AS A CAREER

HEALTHCARE AS A CAREER

INTRODUCTION

This guide was developed to assist healthcare workers at all stages of their careers. The needs of a new graduate healthcare professional are much different than a healthcare worker in his/her fifties giving up direct patient care for less physically demanding work or contemplating retirement. However, issues for all healthcare specialty workers are similar, no matter their age or career phase. This book provides information and resources, allowing healthcare workers to make their own choices. It is designed to be used in tandem with the Introduction to Health Professions, Sixth Edition from Jones and Bartlett Learning. The case studies will allow you to discuss and evaluate situations as you move through your career, or have an event happen to you.

This is a book about self-help, but also about insight into career decisions. I am an independent nurse consultant, which allows me to have many different roles. As a consultant, I am a planner, educator, lecturer, writer, mentor, coach, preceptor and advisor. I use my nursing soul in all these roles.

I have also been the Healthcare Career Expert for Monster.com (2000-2006). In that career advisory role, I was constantly being asked about health-care as a career, and how to deal with issues in the healthcare workforce. I am passionate about nursing and healthcare, and extremely proud of being a nurse. I believe in mentoring and coaching other healthcare workers is part of my responsibility as a professional nurse and a way to be of service. I wanted to create a book that would answer the questions that I have had throughout my career. I also wanted to share what I learned–both good and bad–about navigating my career. Use this book as part of your "career toolkit." As you move through various stages of your career branches, you will face different issues.

While not trained specifically as a career advisor, I believe I have learned things in my thirty seven years as a nurse that may be useful for others. This book does not have all the answers or magic recipes, however, it offers general career advice and concepts that work well in most health careers.

In writing this book, I have learned that how you manage your healthcare career is closely entwined to how you live your life. Self direction, self confidence, spiritual connection in daily life and career development are all part of the same continuum. I hope you find this book helpful.

Overview of the healthcare industry

"Gratitude is the inward feeling of kindness received." This quote is by Henry Van Dyke, and is a wonderful image of the joy working in healthcare professions provides to both caregivers and patients. As one of the largest industries in 2008, healthcare provided 14.3 million jobs for wage and salary workers, according to the Bureau of Labor Statistics (bls.gov). About 40 percent were in hospitals; another 21 percent were in nursing and residential care facilities; and 16 percent were in physician offices.

Currently, even in a tepid economy, ten of the 20 fastest growing occupations are healthcare related (bls.gov). Healthcare will generate 3.2 million new wage and salary jobs between 2008 and 2018, more than any other industry, largely in response to rapid growth in the elderly population. Healthcare jobs can be found throughout the country, but they are concentrated in metropolitan areas.

Health care has been a hot topic among politicians and the public .Many industries will be impacted in some way by new laws, according to Michael Marillo. In some sense everyone will be affected, with some aspects of health care legislation taking effect immediately and others delayed until 2014.

Contained within more than 2,000 pages of new legislation (Affordable Care Act), is the framework for a changing industry, and it will affect both job prospects and job duties . Marillo believes that more insurance and cost coverage will increase demand, especially among boomer age patients. He also believes that electronic medical records will be increasingly significant, and that healthcare jobs will be more ethnically diverse.

There's no question that health care has been a growth industry. The New York Times reported that more than four million people work for hospitals and that hospitals were responsible for hiring 135,000 new employees in 2008. While the economy has impacted most aspects of private business, there are signs that the future looks particularly bright for health care. The new legislation is expected to help as many as 30 million more people obtain coverage over the next few years, which adds to the demand for resources, services, facilities and the administrators needed to oversee them.

Employment in the healthcare industry is projected to increase 22 percent through 2018, compared with 11 percent for all industries combined (bls.gov) Employment growth is expected to account for about 22 percent of all wage and salary jobs added to the economy over the 2008-18 periods. Projected rates of employment growth for the various segments of the industry range from 10 percent in hospitals, the largest and slowest growing industry segment, to 46 percent in the much smaller home healthcare services. (bls.gov)

Healthcare firms employ large numbers of workers in professional and service occupations. Healthcare combines medical technology and human interaction to diagnose, treat, and provide care around the clock, responding to the needs of millions of people—from newborns to the terminally ill (bls.gov). A wide variety of people with various educational backgrounds are necessary for the healthcare industry to function. The healthcare industry employs some highly educated occupations that often require many years of training beyond graduate school. However, many of the occupations in the healthcare industry do not require four years of college.

Professional occupations, such as physicians and surgeons, dentists, registered nurses, social workers, and physical therapists, usually require at least a bachelor's degree in a specialized field or higher education in a specific health field, although registered nurses also may enter through associate degree programs. Professional workers often have high levels of responsibility and complex duties. In addition to providing services, these workers may supervise other workers or conduct research. Some professional occupations, such as medical and health services managers, have limited contact with patients. (bls. gov)

Health technologists and technicians can work in some fast-growing occupations, such as medical records and health information technicians, diagnostic medical sonographers, radiologic technologists and technicians, and dental hygienists. These workers may operate medical equipment and assist a variety of practitioners with diagnosis and/or treatment. These health-care workers typically attend 1-year or 2-year postsecondary (after high school) training programs. (bls.gov) Healthcare service occupations can also attract many workers with minimal or no specialized education or training. Some of these workers are nursing aides, home health aides, building maintenance and cleaning workers, dental assistants, medical assistants, and personal and home care aides.

With many jobs available in the healthcare industry, it is a terrific choice as a second career. Many new graduates of healthcare specialty programs are second career students, entering a nursing or pharmacist program in their mid to late thirties, after working in other, less stable or economically bereft industries like construction or retail. Both Doctor of pharmacy and nursing programs are seeing older students entering these programs as second career options.

Education and Training

A variety of postsecondary programs provide specialized training for jobs in the healthcare industry. People interested in a career as a diagnosing and treating practitioner—such as physicians and surgeons, optometrists, physical therapists, advanced practice nurses or audiologists—should be prepared to complete graduate school coupled with several years of education beyond college. A few healthcare workers need bachelor's degrees like social workers, health service managers, and some registered nurses. A majority of the technologist and technician occupations require a certificate or an associate degree; these programs usually have both classroom and clinical instruction and last about 2 years. Many can be obtained at local community colleges or vocational/technical schools.

Some healthcare facilities provide on-the-job or classroom training, as well as continuing education. Most healthcare workers that do not have postsecondary healthcare training and work directly with patients will receive some on-the-job training. These occupations include nursing aides, orderlies, and attendants; psychiatric aides; home health aides; physical therapist aides; and EKG technicians. Hospitals are more likely than other facilities to have the resources and incentive to provide training programs and advancement opportunities to their employees. In other segments of healthcare, the variety of positions and advancement opportunities are more limited. Larger establishments usually offer a broader range of opportunities. (healthcarejobs.org)

Many hospitals provide training, tuition assistance, or advancement in return for a promise to work at their facility in that role for a particular length of time after graduation. Nursing facilities may have similar programs. Some hospitals have cross-training programs that train their workers—through formal college programs, continuing education, or in-house training—to perform duties outside their specialties.

Opportunities for advancement will vary depending on the occupation itself. Healthcare service assistants and aides may advance to positions with more responsibility with years of experience or additional education or training. Health technologists and technicians often advance by becoming credentialed in a specialty within their field or with additional education or training. Health professionals can also choose to advance to managerial or administrative roles. (healthcarejobs.org)

Should you consider a Healthcare career?

Persons considering careers in healthcare should have a strong desire to help others, genuine concern for the welfare of patients and clients, and an ability to deal with people of diverse backgrounds in stressful situations. Many of the healthcare jobs that are regulated by state licensure require healthcare professionals to complete ongoing continuing education at regular intervals to maintain valid licensure. Before embarking on a health career path, take a few minutes to think about your own abilities, needs, and hopes. The Bureau of Labor and other web sites offer suggestions if you are considering a healthcare career.

Do You Like to Work With People?

How much are you willing to deal with people? Most healthcare roles have constant interactions with a variety of individuals, cultures, and lifestyles. For instance, it is important for nurses, pediatricians, and occupational therapists to have a warm and caring personality. By contrast, other health careers (like medical lab technology, pathology, or medical illustration) involve little or no personal contact with patients.

Do You Like or Do Well in Science?

Many (but not all) health careers require you to be a strong science student. All health careers involve some laboratory science, and some programs demand intensive work in the hard sciences (i.e., chemistry, physics, biology, anatomy, physiology).

Are You Committed to Life Long Learning?

Good health care practitioners are committed to giving their patients the best care available. That means, in order to keep up with the latest developments in your field, you'll need to continue studying and learning throughout your career. Licensed positions have requirements for education content on an ongoing basis.

Are You Comfortable in a Health Care Setting?

Are you prepared to deal with a wide variety of people? In many (but not all) health careers, you may spend much of your time in the company of sick, disabled, or dying people. This will become increasingly common in the near future, as the large "Baby Boomer" generation enters old age. While this opportunity to interact with individuals in some of their most important and intimate moments is an honor, it isn't for everyone. There is an urgent need for health practitioners in medically under-served areas, which often are in rural communities or inner-city neighborhoods.

If you would prefer less direct contact with patients, there are numerous other health-related work settings including pharmacies, laboratories, medical libraries, and corporate, non-profit or government offices that do not require direct patient contact.

Can you work collaboratively as a Team Player?

Health care is a group activity, in which a patient's recovery depends on how well each member of the health care team performs his or her specific function and how well they communicate and collaborate with one another. Even physicians, surgeons and dentist who work in a solo private practice – usually supervise and work closely with several staff members.

What Lifestyle Do You Envision?

How do you feel about facing life-and-death situations on a daily basis? Some (though not all) health careers involve coping with emergencies, working extremely long hours, and shouldering heavy responsibility. What kind of lifestyle do you envision? How much time do you hope to spend at work, versus at home? You need to be realistic and honest with yourself: If you don't mind long workdays and are good at handling stress, go ahead pursue an ER-style career. But if you'd rather have a job with regular hours and fewer medical crises, there are plenty of other fulfilling health careers. No matter what you choose, healthcare is a rewarding career opportunity!

Discussion Questions:
1. Discuss pros and cons of direct patient care jobs you are interested in.
2. Identify three healthcare trends over ten to twenty years.
3. Identify the components of healthcare system.
4. Compare and contrast professional healthcare roles, education and expectations.

Case Studies:
1. Eleanor is a single mother of three small children. She has worked in retail sales until her recent layoff. She is 33 years old. What healthcare careers might she consider? How can she finance any needed education?
2. Fred is a computer programmer who has lost his job twice in 3 years. He knows there has been recent legislation about electronic medical records. He asks your opinion on a healthcare career in this area of specialty. What do you tell him and why?

CAREER DEVELOPMENT

CAREER DEVELOPMENT

Chapter Objectives:

1. Define career development and explain why it is important.
2. Discuss and identify the components of career development.
3. Explain the components of the Turner Career Development model ©.
4. List 5 traits of an indispensable healthcare worker.
5. List 2 methods to improve your career
6. Explain the different types of recruiters and which is most useful to your career choice.

Key terms

Career development   Career enhancement
Career development model   Career self-assessment
Indispensable   Interview
Career plan
Recruiter

Career Development

Career development means taking total responsibility for your career and your life. Career success is not a matter of luck, nor does it just happen–it requires careful planning and analysis. Moving through your career is often thought to be structured like a ladder with different roles at higher and higher levels. In reality, your healthcare career is more like a tree, with many branches and limbs from which to gain experience. Every job and role you take allows you to gather more experience, skills and competencies and place in your career "toolkit". The more tools you have in your tool kit, the more marketable you are.

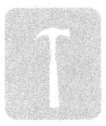 ## For your toolkit... Career success requires careful planning and analysis.

Part of career development includes assessing your educational level. Healthcare is an industry that embraces life-long learning. If you have graduated from a hospital diploma program or a community college program, have you continued your professional learning after graduation? How? It is important to include an educational evaluation in your career assessment. It is important to evaluate what other career options you may have or cannot pursue because you have not enhanced your education level.

Going back to school to earn a bachelor's or master's degree is not for everyone. But, you owe it to yourself to evaluate what it would mean to your career to do so. You can always decide not to go back to school, but at least you have evaluated what education means to you and your career development. If you do decide to go back to school, that additional learning will never be wasted, no matter what career choices you make.

According to Greg Rowlett, you must treat your career like a business and manage it. (2009) Most people do not use good business sense in managing their own careers. Over the years, I have observed that the best students and best managers are not always the most successful in their personal careers. Why? What makes the most difference between success and failure in a career? Is it contacts, luck or plain hard work? All of these components are helpful, but no single specific factor is the determining cause for success or failure.

There are specific things you can do to enhance the chances of success with your career. The first two are crucial, but few people give them any thought. First, choose the right business. Most folks don't recognize the obvious: Whenever you have a choice, choose a great business or organization. Healthcare is a very successful business to be involved in. It is a growing industry with many opportunities for allied health professionals. However, not every healthcare organization is a great one to work in.

Secondly, choose the right strategy. This may seem obvious, but many folks don't consider their own career strategies important. Strategies are the decisions you make to position yourself in a complex environment (Thomas,

1994). Complex environment certainly describes healthcare organization! You must make the choice to manage your strategies actively, or do nothing and let the environment make decisions for you. Doing nothing is never a good idea. Most people mistakenly believe that if they do a good job, they will be successful. Nothing is further from the truth. To be perceived as successful, you must market yourself by differentiating your skills so what you offer is uniquely important to the organization you work in.

You may be wondering how to do this in a healthcare organization when there are many other staff doing exactly the same tasks as you are doing. The answer is to become indispensable. It is not tricky to be perceived by your boss and organization as indispensable. It is all about how you position yourself in the organization and how you are perceived. The traits of an indispensable healthcare professional include the abilities to:

- Demonstrate clinical competence
- Demonstrate leadership skills -planning, coordinating, delegating, supervising the work of others
- Commit and practice life long learning including professional development
- Grasp professional changes in your organization (patient safety focus, increased regulatory and financial requirements)
- Be willing to partner with co workers and your organization to achieve success
- Independence and self direction
- Motivated with high energy
- Objective and non-partisan to special interest mentalities
- Demonstrate integrity
- Demonstrate flexibility and adaptability
- Utilize good time management
- Be assertive and tenacious
- Have a general understanding of JCAHO and other regulatory mandates
- Provide positive role modeling to other staff members

Turner Healthcare Associates, 1998©

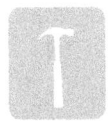 **For your toolkit…Being an indispensable healthcare professional means your skills will always be in demand.**

The third thing that Thomas suggests to increase chances of career success is to develop the right systems. Systems rely on information. Information is crucial for you to be successful. Having the right information at the right time is very important. Many people measure career success by looking at their past performance. This is only part of the picture. As important as it is to look backward, it is more important to look ahead as Wayne Gretsky says, and "go where the puck is."

To get to "where the puck is" you must evaluate skills and abilities of the people at your level in the healthcare industry. What are leaders in your organization and throughout the industry doing to develop themselves and stay ahead of the competition? Read as much as you can and talk to those who know what skills will be required of your specialty in the future. Then you will know how to market yourself.

Fourth, you must design the right career support structure. Individuals need a support structure for their career management. This structure consists of mentors, colleagues, coaches and subordinates to help them achieve objectives. Colleagues and subordinates who can cooperate with you and have complementary skills can be sources for future success. (Thomas, 1994) You can use mentors in your support structure in an active way or passive way. You will likely need both types of mentors in any kind of healthcare career. (See chapter on mentors/coaches) Remember that simply doing a good job does not guarantee success. You must create your own success.

To improve the chance of success in your career:

- Choose a great organization to work for
- Use effective strategies for positioning yourself in the workplace
- Make yourself indispensable, innovative and unique to your organization
- Create effective information loops and support structure
- Enhance all types of communication skills
- Think outside the box about your job and your career

Traits of an Indispensable Healthcare Professional

- Demonstrate clinical competence in your specialty
- Demonstrate leadership skills -planning, coordinating, delegating, supervising the work of others
- Commit and practice life long learning including professional development
- Grasp professional changes in your organization (patient safety focus, increased regulatory and financial requirements)
- Be willing to partner with co workers and your organization to achieve success
- Independence and self direction
- Motivated with high energy
- Objective and non-partisan to special interest mentalities
- Demonstrate integrity
- Demonstrate flexibility and adaptability
- Utilize good time management
- Be assertive and tenacious
- Have a general understanding of JCAHO and other regulatory mandates
- Provide positive role modeling to other staff members

Turner Healthcare Associates, 1998©

As you gain experience as a healthcare professional, you will need to use a career development plan. This plan will have several stages. I created the Turner Career Development Model© while working on my dissertation. You need to critically think through your career path at regular life intervals. I evaluate my situation on my birthday every year. Start by doing an assessment. You can use the Turner Career Self Assessment Tool©, or create your own method. Look at what you are doing and how it is working for you. Complete the assessment and then evaluate your situation. What are you missing in job skills? Are you passionate about your work? Do you want to work as a manager? Once you complete an assessment, then you can create a plan. The Turner Career Development Tool© will assist you in drafting a personal plan for yourself. You must determine how you will get yourself through the transition process that is generated when you make life changes. Take a look at the Turner Transition Model© and the chapter on transition for more information on transition and change.

Last, but not least, evaluate what you have accomplished. Assessment→ Plan→ Manage transition→ Evaluate

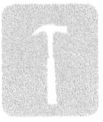

For your toolkit...Assess your career at regular intervals and actively plan your next steps

Turner Career Development Model©

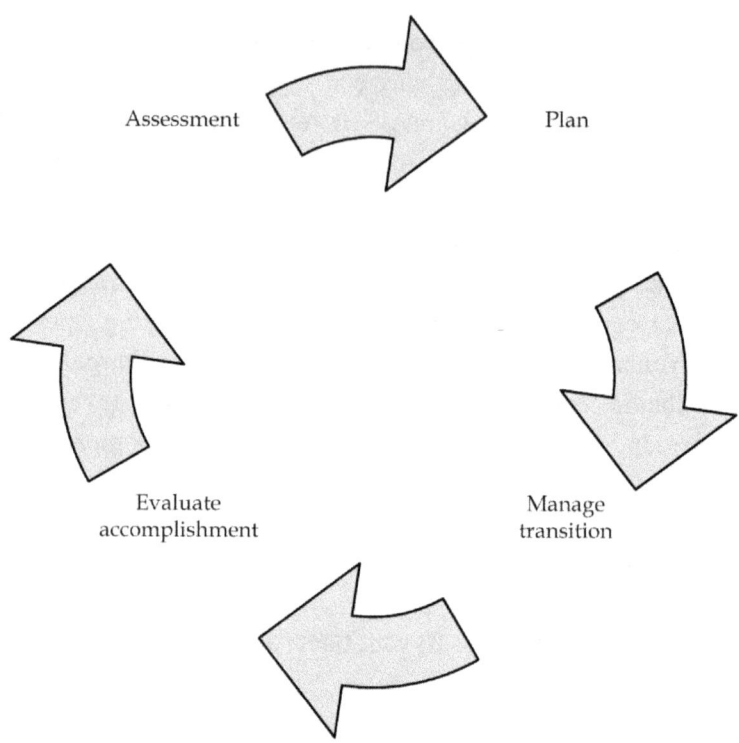

Assessment

Plan

Evaluate
accomplishment

Manage
transition

When we talk with our friends and colleagues about their personal lives and dilemmas, we are often able to see the issues very clearly, even when they cannot. Because we are not emotionally involved in the situation, it makes it easier to sort out the critical issues and determine the best way to proceed to solve the existing problem. That critical thinking process we use with our friends is the same one we need to apply to our own career evaluation. It is always harder to evaluate your own issues, so you may want some help doing this for yourself.

Career development starts with an assessment of where you are and then determining where you want to be. In addition to using the Turner Self Assessment©, planning your personal transition and revitalization, you will also want to create your own plan for the future. To do that, you must implement a career strategy based on critical thinking. It is okay to have more questions than answers. Some other career development tips include:

- Know who to call-trusted friend or mentor

- Think out of the box

- Reach for the stars–anything goes

- Use the assessment tool to create short and long term goals

- Evaluate income needs vs. personal satisfaction

- Be a risk taker

- Consider more education

- Believe you can do whatever you want to be successful

To get started, you can choose experts to assist you at different aspects of your career. Make your planning and managing multifaceted. Be sure to include both your life responsibilities and your career in your assessment. You may want to set new goals with yourself and your manager as you move through the assessment process.

Assess your educational level and future educational needs and update your resume annually. Create personal one year and five year plans for your career. Identify steps and strategies to implement your career plan. Evaluate what you enjoy and are good at. Assess why you love your work. It is important to determine early on if you are going to work at a profession you love or are you going to a job?

Healthcare professionals must be active in their own career development. Many simply move from job to job without considering long term strategies or career goals. This can lead to stagnation and burn out. Before you begin, take stock of where you are in your present job. Are you doing your best? Are you enthusiastic? Burned out? Bored? There are numerous texts on how to evaluate your career, but the one I like best is the *Graduate Handbook of Job Searching Techniques.* (Stern) I have adapted that process for my Turner Career Development Assessment Tool©

Start by evaluating your present role. Taking stock of where you are is the most important step of your career planning process. To avoid making choices blindly, you must find out where you are, what you have to offer, and how you fit into the big-and rapidly changing- health care industry. Read. Listen. Watch. Learn. Find out as much as you can about the national and local trends in healthcare. This will tell you what the future opportunities will be. The more insight you have, the better equipped you will be to handle the changes.

It is important to design a future for yourself that is a good fit for you and where you are at different stages of life. In their twenties and thirties, most folks have big dreams and make long range plans. Once you hit your forties, the ideas change to what makes you happy NOW. It is easy to get caught in the assumption that we are somehow set apart from the passing of time.

We always assume that we can do all the things we dream of doing. We just don't have time to do them now. We perceive that our life will somehow be automatically better, and that sometime in the far distant future we will, be nicer and finally do things like lose 40 pounds, learn to play the twelve string guitar and write in a journal.

When you are living the overwhelming grind of working *towards* your future, you end up thinking that you can always do your wish list someday. Suddenly someday is *NOW*. When you look at where you are going, the future needs to fit who you are becoming. If you are young, realize that your future will change as you age and you will be making this assessment again.

The future when you are 40 is not the same as when you were younger. Besides financial planning (a MUST!) for your older years, you must also imagine a future from where you are. You need to take an honest look at your life and figure out what future fits where you are now. You need to start the process of creating a future that fits the person you are becoming-not one that fits who you have been. As Ronna Lichtenberg suggests, you can write a working scenario and a not-working scenario. Describe it in great detail–who is there, what kind of work or activities you are doing, what you are wearing (2005). Make two scenarios. Consider the best possible future and your worst possible future. Make the scenario, and then put it away. Give yourself at least a week, and then find time to review both your best– and worst– future versions. Identify with what feels like a big deal to you in both scenarios. Find the clues for what you really want to have in your future that is a change from how you are living your life now. (Lichtenberg, 2005)

Once you know this, you can create your action plan. Start with one thing you can do that will take you toward the future you want to have. Your future doesn't have to be black and white answers. It can have "maybes" also. Maybe you can try something different. Maybe you can change jobs. Doing this exercise will help remind you that you are here–now–and that your old future may not fit anymore. You will discover that you are still a work in progress, and that is a good thing.

After you have written your best and worst future scenarios, evaluate what they look like. Consider your present job. What do you like? Dislike? What are you good at? Not so good at? Think about what makes you happy in your work. Be honest. Next, think about what you would like and not like in a job. Travel? Management responsibility? Flexible scheduling? Children? Healthy people? Old people? Inmates? Think about all the issues and be open-minded. Thinking "outside the box" gives you more ways to put together something that will work just right for your life.

Gather information about roles you like. Look on the web, at advertisements in healthcare journals and talk to colleagues about what their jobs entail. Once you have lots of information, you can choose one or two roles that you want to pursue. Find out all you can about these roles. Make sure they fit will with your professional goals and your personal life. Decide on a role to pursue, and find out about educational requirements, salary, training required and job availability. Consider job shadowing for a day with someone already in the role you are looking into.

Next, you need to plan your strategies. Talk with your current supervisor about your plans. Chances are s/he will support you. Investigate when you can attend school, change your schedule or rearrange child care to pursue your interest. Make sure you consider all the possibilities. Be flexible in your approach and also make a back-up plan for each strategy.

Once you have planned your strategies, you need to implement them. This is easier said than done. You actually have to DO things–not just talk or read about them. This is where to put your energy into moving forward with your plan. Make sure your supervisor, co-workers, and significant others know you are working towards a professional goal and will need their support and understanding. Most of the time you will find everyone to be supportive. Don't forget to include arrangements for child care during class time, time for class reading or to write papers when you are implementing your plan.

Continue your career management throughout your professional life. Pick a date and assess where you are annually. I usually use my birthday, and determine whether I like where I am professionally and what I want to do differently. To do this on an ongoing basis, you must acknowledge your own needs and changing life issues. If you have small children, what you can tolerate professionally is different than when your children are fully grown.

As with other life assessments, be sure you also consider what you cannot do and what you are not. This sounds odd, but you need to be honest about what you cannot do, so you don't set yourself up to get into a job situation where you do that particular skill all the time. In my case, I would never want a job or role that requires lots of budgeting and financial skills. I can read and manage budgets just fine, but don't want to spend any of my time crunching numbers. I am lousy at math, and therefore need to include that challenge in my career planning. I also get bored easily. I need changing activities to stay passionate about my work. Knowing your limitations are as important as knowing your strengths! Identify what you need to deal with those limitations. In my case, it means using a really good calculator all the time and resource people with financial skills.

As you continue to manage your career, be sure you assess where you want to be in the future as well as right now. What do you want to do in two years? In five? What is your personal mission statement? Use the Turner Career Self Assessment Tool © to create your own personal career plan. Understanding these things about your self is crucial to accurate career planning. Talk to your mentors regularly, but no less than once a year. Reward yourself for actually implementing your career plan as well as successes. It is easy to get bogged down in the details of what you are currently doing. Don't forget what your long term and future goals are.

More Career development tips:

- Work at your own level of professional development
- Evaluate your own clinical/specialty performance
- Direct your own professional and career growth
- Pursue your own professional interests and specialties
- Receive objective competency-based performance evaluations focused on the nursing process and leadership skills
- Decide whether you want to work toward advancing your expertise or preparing for future roles.
- Decide whether higher education will enhance your role performance.
- Complete job self assessment/stress assessment/skills inventory
- Explore roles that interest you
- Gather information about the roles that interest you (the education, training, and skills required)
- Target the roles you are most interested in
- Make a decision about the role you will pursue first
- Strategize about how you will achieve that role
- Implement your strategy
- Reward yourself for your success
- Manage your career regularly and no less than annually (on your birthday or another day each year)

Discussion Questions:

1. Discuss pros and cons of career development
2. Identify 3 characteristics/methods to improve your career.
3. Identify 4 components of Turner Career Development model and explain each one.
4. Compare and contrast the types of recruiters and their importance to your career choices.

5. Identify 3 interview questions and your answers to them.

6. List two ways you can enhance your career.

7. Have each student complete self-assessment documents. Discuss in small groups to identify trends or issues.

8. Discuss components of a successful interview process

Case Studies:

1. Alex is a housekeeper in a community hospital. He is married with 5 children. He has worked in this role at the same facility for 20 years. He is interested in a career that will pay more, have less physical demands and will provide a good retirement. How would you assist him?

2. A recruiter calls you to ask if you would be interested in a job as a manager in your area of expertise. It is an existing role in a competing facilities What questions would you ask the recruiter? Why?

 **Turner Career Self Assessment Tool©**

1. The tasks and components I like most about my present job are:

2. The tasks and components I like least about my present job are:

3. The tasks I excel in at in my present job are:

4. The tasks I struggle with in my present job are:

5. My education goals are:

6. My life long learning goals are:

7. My short term (within one year) goal (s) is (are): By 20___ , I will have:

8. The steps I need to take to achieve this short term goal are:

9. My long term (two to three years) goal (s) is (are): By 20___, I will have:

10. The steps I need to take to achieve this long term goal are:

11. Jobs outside the acute care hospital that interest me are:

12. Areas of cross training or specialization within the hospital that interest me are:

13. The resources I need to achieve my short term and long term goals are:

Turner Healthcare Associates, Inc, ©1994

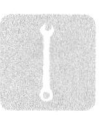 **Turner Career Development Assessment Tool©**

1. What are you doing now? Describe your work and role:

2. What do you want and need in a job and role? (list points from the self assessment tool)

3. Gather information about the roles you like: what do you know about these roles? What do you like about them? What else can you find out? Where? When?

4. Target one or two roles to aim for: What is it? Where is it done? Who do you know that you could job shadow in this role?

5. Decide which one role you actually want to do. If you had to make a decision today, what would you choose? Why?

6. List and explain four strategies to achieve the role you chose in the previous question.

7. To implement your strategies you would have to do what? How? When? Where?

8. Is furthering your professional education important to you? Why or why not?

9. If you want to further your professional education, what will you do? When? How?

10. Decide on a method for you to continue your ongoing career development and management. What will the method include? When will you do it?

11. How will you know you are successful at achieving your goal(s)? List your criteria for success.

12. What will you do to reward yourself for your success? When?

Turner Healthcare Associates, Inc. © 1994

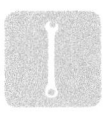 **Turner Career Planning Process©**

1. Where do you want to be in 3-5 years?
2. What do you want and like in a job?
3. Gather information about the roles you like. List them.
4. Target 1-2 roles to aim for. List them.
5. Decide on 1 role to do. List it.
6. Develop 5 strategies to achieve that role (school, certification, job shadow).
7. Implement your 5 strategies, one at a time.
8. Evaluate your outcomes and continue ongoing career management.

Turner Healthcare Associates, Inc, © 1994

 **Turner Stress Assessment Tool ©**

For the purposes of this test, stress is defined as a mismatch between the demands placed on you and your ability to meet those demands.

Circle the correct response for you. There are no "right" answers!

1. Do you feel stressed at work?   Yes   No

2. Do you feel more stressed at work now than you did three years ago?
   Yes   No

3. Do you feel more stressed at work now than you did one year ago?
   Yes   No

4. How stressed to you feel right now?   Not at all   Not much
   Fairly   Some   Very

5. If you feel stressed how does this manifest itself? Circle all that apply:

Physically

Headaches   stomach/bowel problems   chest pain   frequent
infections   sleep problems   weight loss   weight gain   loss of libido

Psychological

Moodiness/irritability   tiredness   apathy   depression   anxiety
Frustration   indecision   boredom   feeling guilty   poor concentration

Behaviorally

Accident-prone   alcohol abuse   drug abuse   food abuse
Aggressiveness   relationship difficulties   absenteeism

6. How do you feel stress in your personal life affect you at work?
   Not at all   a little   quite a bit   a lot

7. How do you feel stress at work affects your personal life?

    Not at all   a little   quite a bit   a lot

8. If you feel stressed, what would you say are the major causes of your stress?

    Excessive workload   lack of resources   staff-related

    Management- related   patient-related   personal difficulties

    Changes within profession   job insecurity   job transition/new job

9. How do you cope with stress?

    Counseling   support groups   recreational activities   relaxation

    Stress management techniques   talking with friends/significant other

    Regular exercise   alcohol/drugs/nicotine/food

    missing work   denial

10. How would you rate your ability to cope with stress?

    Poor   Average   Better than average   Very good

11. How many stress-related sick leave/days have you used in the past year?

Turner Healthcare Associates, Inc © 1994

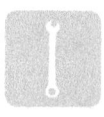 ## Turner Indispensable Assessment Tool ©

Are you in a position of being indispensable to your boss or unit? Take this assessment to see how indispensable you are. The more yes answers you have, the more indispensable you are!

1. Are you clinically/specialty competent?
2. Do you have general understanding of JCAHO accreditation and requirements?
3. Do you have general understanding of managed care/payor issues that affect your geographic area?
4. Do you have general understanding of budget and cost issues that affect your facility?
5. Are you willing to be a partner with your institution, not just an employee?
6. Do you have decision making skills?
7. Are you self directed, not always expecting to be told what to do?
8. Do you have integrity?
9. Do you have an objective perspective?
10. Do you act like a victim?
11. Do you have a strong work ethic? (not a workaholic)
12. Do you have a high energy level?
13. Do you have effective time management skills?
14. Do you have a strong positive self image?
15. Do you have effective interpersonal skills
16. Are you flexible?
17. Are you excited, not threatened by change?
18. Can you deal with change and get mobilized, even if you are afraid?
19. Are you adaptable?
20. Are you assertive?

21. Are you tenacious?

22. Do you have personal ambition and drive?

23. Are you self-motivated and a self-starter?

Turner Healthcare Associates, Inc. ©1998

Resumes

Having a winning (not just acceptable) resume is the beginning to finding your first job. When human resource staff and recruiters receive hundreds of resumes a day, the best strategy to narrow down the "keepers" is through the process of elimination.

Your resume becomes the only tool to let your reader know why you would be the right person for the job. You need to create a useful resume.

There are zillions of books available on how to create a resume. You can purchase one, consult on-line experts at locations like Monster.com, or hire someone to create a resume for you. No matter how you choose to create your resume, here are the most crucial things to remember.

A resume *must* be free of spelling errors, typos and poor grammar. Always include a cover letter that speaks specifically to the job you are applying for. Use appropriate and professional formatting. Make the resume no longer than two pages. Use bullet points, not long paragraphs. When listing experience versus education, list the heading first where you have spent the most time recently. Be sure you have a resume that explains what your accomplishments were and how you achieved them, not just a listing of job descriptions or tasks. Make sure your employer hiring dates and contact information is accurate and complete. Do not list personal information that is irrelevant to the job you are applying for. Your height, weight, marital status, GPA and other personal information do not belong in a professional resume. List your previous employment in chronological order. Explain any gaps in your employment in the cover letter, not in the resume. Be honest about your education, titles, training and salary. It can be devastating to lie on your resume and get caught. I discuss the ramification of this in the chapter on professional advocacy.

When you write a cover letter, include the date, your name and contact information. List a contact person's name, title and address. Take the time to find this out to send a personal cover letter. Add an appropriate salutation. Stay away from "Dear Sir/Madam," as it is too impersonal. State the reason and purpose for your contact and correspondence. Express your interest in a position or working at that facility. List your qualifications, experiences and education that makes you the right candidate for the job.

Identify and address any red flags in your resume. If you have gaps in work history, have relocated or left a job, address those briefly in your cover letter. Make a philosophical statement about what you bring to the job you are interested in or why you became a nurse. State an action step you will take. Identify what you will do next, e.g. call next week. Be proactive about getting an interview and call the facility to set one up unless it is specifically stated that the facility does not want to receive calls.

Interviews

Your mother was right. First impressions really do matter. As has often been said, you never get a second chance to make a first impression. First impressions in job interviews usually make or break the rest of the process. Healthcare is a job seeker's paradise. Even so, workers should not assume that jobs are always available, or that they "landed the job" after a pleasant interview. Believing that the job is automatically yours because of the large number of vacant positions is risky. I was even shown my office at a job I thought sure I got–and then found out they hired someone else! Landing a job requires more than just showing up. Interview techniques and expectations have evolved and the strategies you used twenty years ago won't work anymore. Preparation for an interview is now the most important thing you can do to be successful.

 **For your toolkit... First impressions in job interviews make or break the rest of the process.**

Most healthcare interviews now include questions based on a behavioral-based model (case scenarios). These kinds of questions cannot be answered with a simple yes or no. Behavioral questions are designed to glean specific explanations of scenarios from interviewees and how they react to a given situation. How applicants answer the questions is as important as what they say. These type of questions are designed to get an interviewee to describe a circumstance that has happened in their past work environment and how they dealt with it. The idea behind these types of questions is that the best predictor of future behavior is past behavior. Be sure to evaluate scenarios in your career that you can speak to. Those situations that involve conflict resolution, impressive communication strategies or major contributions are the ones to mention during the interview.

Don't forget to do your homework. Remember, you are interviewing the facility as much as they are interviewing you. You need to research the institution to learn about any specialty areas, the care philosophy, and any specifics about the unit or area you are interviewing for. Arriving prepared for an interview sends the message that you are interested in the facility as much as they are interested in you.

Also, there are several generations active in professional healthcare roles. As Jennifer Hermann, Director of Workplace Planning at UCSF Medical Center, says, "That is a huge age range for ideas, attitudes and expectations." Many people doing interviews are in their forties and fifties. They may have very different perceptions on work related issues than a new grad under thirty. Remember to pay attention to how you are dressed and how you conduct yourself. This will minimize chances for miscommunication. Hermann believes that taking a more formal approach when being interviewed by someone like this can show respect for their view of the profession. (Cowle, 2005)

Doing Your Interview Homework-Prepare for the interview

Be sure you can answer the following questions prior to going to the interview:

- Will I be effective with my skills/abilities working with this employer?
- Are there jobs available in roles I am interested in and qualified for?
- How does this employer treat employees?
- Is this employer financially stable?
- What are the opportunities for advancement? For women/minorities?

- How does this organization rank within the healthcare industry?
- What are the services offered by this organization?
- Does this organization have problems that my skills can help solve?
- How do employees that work in this organization feel about their jobs?
- What is the turnover of employees in this organization?
- How does this organization communicate with employees? Externally?
- Does this organization encourage professional development and advancement? Provide scholarships or tuition reimbursement?
- What kind of management style does the person have that I would report to? Does it blend with my personality and professional characteristics?
- Do I know what the job description requirements/tasks are?

(Adapted from Nurses Guide to Managed Care, 1996)

How to Create a Successful Interview

Preparing in advance can help lower your stress level and improve your performance during the process. Research the company to learn as much as you can and make sure it is the right environment for you. Read the facility's mission statement, core values, where its' focus is and some recent successes or achievements. Use and speak about the researched information to demonstrate your knowledge and interest during the interview. Rehearse the interview. Practice your facial expression, eye contact, handshake and body language. Practice answering likely interview questions so you don't stumble over the wording.

When planning your schedule, allow at least two hours for the interview. In some cases, you'll actually need an entire day. Professionals dress professionally: Men usually wear ties, dress shoes and a sports coat. Women wear blue or black suits, hosiery and dress shoes. Check yourself in a full length mirror, front *and* back, before you leave your residence. Avoid displaying anything that may take attention away from your skills and qualifications trendy fashions, tattoos, nose rings, intense makeup, etc. Arrive at the interview a few minutes early. Always make sure you allow extra time if you are unfamiliar with the location.

Be polite. Show respect to everyone you meet, no matter whether it's the boss, the receptionist or a prospective coworker. Shake hands firmly and make eye contact with the interviewer. Know what questions you should answer and what questions are illegal (age, marital status, children, race, religion, sexual preferences or personal habits). Focus your comments on what you can offer the facility to solve its' problems.

Be familiar with your work history and skills. Explain gaps in employment and why you left past jobs. Frame these comments in a positive way. Try and recall specific work situations or scenarios when answering questions. Bring a resume with you. Even if the interviewer has a copy, another can be useful for you to reference as you answer questions.

Gather information and bring it with you. Phone numbers, addresses of past employers, employment dates, etc. Bring license and certifications and specialty training cards (e.g. ACLS). Do not write "see resume" on the application. Bring a neatly typed list of professional references. Include the relationship of the reference to you and the best way to reach that person. Be sure to contact each person you list as a reference *before* you give the list to an interviewer, so your references will not be surprised or uncomfortable about getting a call from a facility.

Think of yourself as a product with features and benefits you want to sell, and gear your answers accordingly. Focus on what the interviewer really wants to know. Identify your job skill features. How will your features benefit this employer? Healthcare workers definitely need good people skills. However, another prerequisite of the job is a measure of technical literacy. Be confident about your skills and explain how your experiences and interests are a match for the position.

Be comfortable talking about your self. Confidence and enthusiasm are critical characteristics of an interview. Prepare three to five questions to ask the interviewer. Asking insightful questions sets you apart from the rest of the pack of applicants. Questions demonstrate that you've done your homework about the company, and that you are as interested in finding out how you'll fit in and achieve your career goals as they are in learning whether you're the right person for the job. Ask specific questions about the position: to whom you will report, job expectations, how they manage people, what the greatest challenge is in the job

Never ask about salary, vacation or other benefits during a job interview. The time to talk about money and benefits is after the employer has offered you the job.

Follow up with a thank-you letter to the interviewer or a phone call to communicate your interest in the position and to follow up on any additional questions you need to answer. In your letter be sure you address that:

- You heard what specifics the interviewer mentioned about the role
- You are excited about the job, can do the job and want the job
- You have excellent communication skills and will mesh well with the organization
- You clear up any confusion, negative impressions or provide clarifications.

Most recruiters agree that the person who gets the job is not always the most qualified, but they usually know how to prepare and do the best interview. Always keep in mind that basic interview protocols never go out of style. A formal interview approach, professional business attire, and a personal, handwritten thank you note to follow up are always appropriate and will isolate you above other jobseekers. Everything you do to obtain a new position, including written communication and how you dress, needs to indicate that you are highly professional. Remember that the small things can make a really big difference.

Working with a Recruiter

Many hard to find, middle management and senior executive positions are filled by corporate recruiters. This means that the facility with the job hires a recruiter to find and screen qualified job candidates. A recruiter's job is to provide a pool of qualified candidates for open positions and to help the hiring manager choose the most qualified candidate from that pool to fill the job requisition. There are several types of recruiters and it helps to know the difference. In almost all but the rarest cases, recruiters represent the hiring entity, not the candidate.

AGENCY RECRUITERS: Agencies recruiters can work independently be associated with a small "boutique" firm that focuses on a particular industry, or be part of a large firm. Agency recruiters can fill either full-time or temporary positions, but their compensation always comes as the direct result of filling a position for a client company. If it's a temp position, the agency gets a mark-up over the hourly rate to cover statutory taxes, any benefits offered and paid for by the client company, and the agency's profit margin. If it's a full-time regular position, then compensation usually happens in one of two ways– contingency placement or retained search.

With a contingency placement, the agency is paid only when a candidate is hired (and often completes their probationary period). A client company might ask multiple agencies to work on one search and then hire the best candidate. Agencies will work on contingency positions if and only if they think they have a good chance of filling the position in a short amount of time, otherwise the efforts exceed the rewards. Contingency searches are usually employed for positions where there's a large candidate pool for any one position.

On a retained search, the agency is paid a fee to fill a position and they work on the search until the position is filled. The fee is generally paid in installments– usually 1/3 up front, 1/3 upon presentation of 3 qualified candidates, and 1/3 upon candidate placement. The agency is also usually reimbursed for all of their expenses, including travel to interview candidates. Retained searches are usually used for professional level positions only, and almost always at the management and executive level.

EXECUTIVE RECRUITERS: Executive search firms (technically agencies but they don't like to be called that!) specialize in filling positions at the management and executive level. They rarely get involved with temp work or temp positions. Almost all of their work is handled on a retained search basis.

RESEARCH FIRMS: Executive search firms and other agencies often employ research firms (sometimes their own) to identify potential candidates for positions. Sometimes it's the research firms that make initial contact with a candidate and the recruiter actually takes over at a later point in the process.

CORPORATE RECRUITERS: Also called in-house recruiters, corporate recruiters are employed by one company and work on behalf of that company to find qualified candidates to fill the company's positions. Corporate recruiters are generally paid as salaried employees or hourly contractors, although they can sometimes receive bonuses for filling positions.

When you're speaking with a recruiter it pays to know what type of recruiter they are – corporate, agency, research, executive search, etc. You should be comfortable asking them about their role and where they are in the search process. Before giving your resume to an agency you should find out (and even get in writing) exactly where they intend to submit your resume. Once your resume has been submitted to a company through an agency you may be unable to submit your resume on your own for some period of time. If the client really wasn't an actual client but just a "potential" client you may be left in a stalemate situation with an employer who wants to interview you and can't or won't pay the agency fee.

When contacted by a recruiter you should also ask if he or she is calling about a specific opportunity, a future opportunity, or general career opportunities with a particular employer. If it's an executive search agency and they have a current search for which you're a fit, then it's a serious conversation. If they've seen your resume on a job board and think you might be a fit for upcoming positions at one or more client firms, then the conversation isn't quite so serious.

Some candidates think of recruiters as roadblocks. That isn't the case! Recruiters want to fill the position and will always look for ways to rule a candidate "in" rather than rule a candidate 'out'. Recruiters are like "sellers" agents in real estate – they work for the company, not for the candidate. Candidates sometimes forget this and think it's a recruiter's responsibility to find them a job or to give them career advice.

The hiring process is very time intensive. With the advent of internet job sites, email, company web sites, a recruiter can receive hundreds of resumes a day. They will pay more attention to resumes that are well-written (no typos) and easy to read. Candidates should do their best to make their resumes attractive to an employer. Explain gaps in job history, if you've made lots of job changes. Also state if you're willing to relocate, if you've just relocated, etc. You can use a cover letter or summary section to highlight skills specific to a position. It's unlikely that a recruiter will have time to go back and ask you for clarification. "When I received a cover letter addressed to a competitor instead of my company I didn't even look at the resume but immediately rejected the candidate," remarked Sutzi McGovern MBA, a self employed technical recruiter. "Another resume I rejected without even reviewing stated an objective of a product manager when the position they applied for was a software engineer. This indicates to me that the candidate is not detail oriented. While this may not be the case and they may just be pushed for time, they lost my attention."

Certain positions have very specific requirements or budget constraints. Even if you're the brightest new grad on the planet a recruiter won't be able to hire you for a senior-level position, and vice versa. If the position is budgeted for a junior-level hire, they can't fill it with someone earning twice as much, even if you're willing to take a position with less responsibility.

Most recruiters always assume that candidates are on their "best" behavior during the interview process and that any behavioral "red flags" uncovered during the interviews will only be magnified once you start work. Recruiters are a key player in employers' decision making process so please treat them with respect and be considerate of their time. Here are some typical questions about recruiters and the answers I received from both healthcare and high tech recruiters.

How do I find a recruiter?

If a candidate cold calls, that starts the ball rolling. Depending on time and their communication skills, a recruiter may try to determine right then and there if there is a current appropriate match. If there is a match, the recruiter will ask them to email a resume. After it is reviewed by the recruiter, a decision is made whether it fits any current positions. If so, it is forwarded to a manager and the candidate is informed that a referral has occurred. If there is no match, the candidate knows that as well. If it's a resume where there would be future interest, it will likely be stored in a tickler file.

If you want to meet a recruiter, how do you find one?

McGovern, with over 15 years in recruiting with such firms as Cisco Systems, Inc, Nokia and Farmers Insurance Group, suggests asking friends or family. McGovern gives an example of a missed networking opportunity. "One of my best friends, Pat, was recently attending an open house. She told me the name of the recruiter who contacted her and it was a former colleague of mine, Cynthia, who I know very well. I told Pat this and specifically told her to tell Cynthia that she and I were friends. I asked Pat how the event was. She said, "Cynthia was so busy that all I had time to do was shake her hand." All Pat needed to do when she was shaking hands is say, "By the way I'm a good friend of Sutzi's," and Cynthia would have remembered her and sent me an email asking about her. Now she is just one of hundreds who shook hands with the recruiter. Ask friends who placed them in particular jobs. Go to job fairs to meet corporate recruiters. Call into a company and ask to speak with someone in recruiting. Generally, though, recruiters will come find you. Never pay for a recruiter. It is acceptable to pay to have your resume done professionally, but it's really not necessary unless you can't type and have no access to a computer or printer. Some websites have the recruiters' email addresses. It doesn't hurt to send a resume even if there is not an exact match at the time, especially if it's a company you are targeting.

How do you know if a recruiter is reputable?

Ask them for references. Check the internet. Trust your gut. If they seem slimy, they probably are! Agency recruiting is sales, just like cars, real estate, insurance, except that both our clients and our products are people. Other candidates will be able to tell you and there are reputable recruiters working for companies that may not be reputable. If they know someone in a job they want ask that person how they got the job.

Do recruiters give career/resume/interview advice to you?

It depends on the recruiters' volume of work. McGovern says, "If I have the time, I do all of the above." "If I have developed a rapport (usually by doing a phone interview) with them and think they may be a match I will give them interview hints." " If I see it's just naiveté on their part, I do give them resume advice even if I'm not bringing them in for an interview."

Some corporate recruiters want to see how a candidate does on their own without coaching. An executive recruiter on a retained search has the luxury of a longer hiring cycle and also has more at stake, so might spend considerable time coaching an executive candidate on who they'll be meeting and what the hiring managers are looking for. An executive recruiter will also likely rewrite your resume to put in a presentation-style format. Many recruiters will be happy to answer questions from candidates about who they'll be meeting, what to wear for the interview, etc. You should also ask questions of the recruiter and the hiring manager about the company and especially about what the key success factors for this particular position and/or employer are. The answers should give you some big clues as to what topics might be covered in an interview.

Should you ask a recruiter for their input on a specific job?

It is okay to ask any recruiter about the position. However, most of them aren't necessarily familiar with the specifics of the position or the technical aspects of a particular job - that's for the hiring manager ad others on the team to discuss.

Should you contact a recruiter if you hear about a job you want?

Different companies have different rules about letting candidates through. It is always a good idea to try, especially with corporate recruiters. If you are dealing with an agency recruiter, contact them only if you are certain that a particular agency or search firm is doing the hiring for the position you want.

Is recruiting at the executive/senior management level any different that at the mid management/director level?

Definitely. At the executive level there is almost always an executive search firm involved. And, as a rule, the hiring process takes longer the higher up you go in an organization. The candidates are usually known entities that are being convinced to join a company. There is more wooing then because the candidates have a known track record. If you're working with an executive search firm you might have multiple interviews with the recruiter and/or research firm before even being presented as a candidate to the client.

Should a recruiter make comments about whether you should take a job or not?

Most recruiters discuss with a candidate whether this is the right job for them. It may be more the company culture that may not match or a certain manager. Some recruiters believe it's a two way street and the company and job should be right for the candidate also. Whether you are working with a corporate or agency recruiter, the client is usually the employer, not the candidate. Candidates should know what's important to them in a job and do their best to ask appropriate questions during the interview process in order to determine their fit with a particular employer and/or position. McGovern adds "As a corporate recruiter I do believe it's a two way street and the company and job should be right for the candidate. I also believe that if a candidate is encouraged to take a job that is not a fit (for whatever reason) it can lead to poor performance and possible termination.

It's most important for a corporate recruiter to assist with the right fit as this affects their long term relationship with the hiring manager and ultimately could affect whether they keep their assignment and/or get rehired in the future. An agency recruiter would take a chance that the poor performance wouldn't manifest until after they were paid. They go from client to client and most have no relationship with the hiring manager but with the recruiting department instead." "In this economy I know some candidates are desperate and will take any job but it will look worse on their resume if they have a short term stint and are fired then if they were never hired in the first place, says McGovern."

Is it appropriate to work around a recruiter and talk directly to facility staff?

Usually what happens is the staff member will forward the resume or place a phone call to the recruiter. Very rarely will a candidate get an interview this way. If the candidate is a friend or family member of an executive or senior management, they may be given a courtesy interview but this is very rare. Unless you've been told otherwise by a recruiter or by someone on the staff, I think its okay to use your personal contacts within an organization to try to find a job. But once you've been told that you need to deal with the recruiter, you need to do so.

What if a recruiter tells you a job is one thing and it is actually something else?

Let the recruiter know that his or her information was incorrect about the position. Sometimes it's not the recruiter's fault that the information is bad - sometimes the employer hasn't given out the best information or there might have been a miscommunication during the interview process. The interview should give you the best idea of the job. It's always good practice even if the job isn't right for the candidate. Also sometimes the criteria change from when the interview was scheduled until the interview is actually conducted.

What if you are recruited and the job is a bad fit?

Talk to your manager or the recruiter. Depending on how long it's taken the candidate to realize the bad fit, there may be something that can be done. If it's because of performance issues, the candidate may be let go. With a corporate recruiter, they have to go back and fill the position again. Agency contracts usually have a replacement clause where a portion of the fee is refunded or a replacement candidate is provided.

How is the recruiter affected?

Unless every candidate turns out not to be a good fit, not much happens. In most companies, the final decision to hire is with the manager and their team.

If they are making a lot of bad hires, the recruiter usually steps in and does some interview training or assesses what the real issues are with the Human Resources partner.

How are recruiters paid?

Corporate recruiters are paid a salary no matter how many hires they create. If they don't meet goals, that is reflected in their performance review. If they are on contract, it may not be renewed. Agency recruiters are either contingency or retained. If they are contingency they get a specified percentage of the gross salary after the candidate has been employed; usually 90 days. Retained are usually for executive search and they have contracts that pay them a certain amount during all the different stages of the search.

Should you talk to recruiters even if you aren't looking for a job?

If contacted by a recruiter you should always be gracious because you never know when you'll need their services. Get their name and number and keep them on file for the future. If they pester you, tell them not to call– they're probably not someone you want to work with anyway. If you're not interested in a particular position but know someone who is, give them that person's name or take their name to give to their friend. Recruiting is all about networking and what you put out there can come back to help you in a very big way. If you talk to them when you don't want to they are more likely to remember and will talk to you when you need a job. That day always comes. Also you may be able to refer a friend who's looking for a job and that's a win-win.

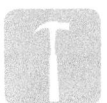 **For your toolkit…Create a relationship with at least one recruiter. You never know when you will need one!**

NOTE: The author wishes to acknowledge and thank the recruiter who assisted her with developing this chapter. Sutzi McGovern provided invaluable information and insight.

ENCOURAGING OTHERS TO SUCCEED: MENTORING, COACHING, AND PRECEPTING OTHERS

"An Expert was once a Beginner"
-Dr. Patricia Benner

ENCOURAGING OTHERS: MENTORING, COACHING, AND PRECEPTING

Chapter Objectives:

1. Define and explain mentoring.
2. Define and explain coaching and why it is necessary.
3. Compare and contrast the differences between coaching and mentoring.
4. Explain the role of preceptor and why it is important to new healthcare workers.

Key terms

Coaching   Mentoring

Preceptor

Effective Mentoring

All healthcare professional have a need for special insight, understanding, wisdom and information that a mentor or executive coach can provide. Coaches and mentors can help individuals successfully navigate multiple challenges, changes and demands. The need for coaching and mentoring has never been more apparent for leaders at all levels, because how people progress within their careers is changing. (Gates, 2004)

Webster's defines mentoring as a trusted counselor or guide, tutor or coach, preceptor or teacher (9th edition). According to Hein and Nicholson, "mentoring occurs when a senior person (the mentor) in terms of age and/or experience, undertakes to provide information, advice and emotional support for a junior person in a relationship lasting over an extended period of time and marked by substantial emotional commitment by both parties." (Gates, 2004)

Examples of mentoring include any healthcare student with an experienced provider, a new manager with an experienced manager or orientation of a new employee with a "buddy." There is a difference between mentoring and precepting. Precepting is a formal role, and is covered in a separate section.

Mentoring is not power driven, authoritarian "my way or no way" or punitive. Mentoring is not something you are mandated to do in your career—forced compliance is not required. Mentoring is something you chose to do, and you accept the mentee completely, without judgment of his or her choices or behaviors.

Healthcare professionals interested in mentoring usually like sharing what they know. They are willing to teach and enjoy working with students, new grads and new employees. They willingly accept the time commitment to work with mentees. Successful mentors are able to evaluate outcomes, be kind, fair, empathetic and objective. They are willing to share their own good and bad experiences, because "Good judgment comes from experience. Experience comes from bad judgment." (Unknown source) Mentors can assess how mentees best learn and provide praise and supportive criticism. Mentors are willing to influence others and to stretch and push mentees to grow and learn. They help mentees develop a realistic picture of themselves and their skills.

There is an interface between mentoring, professionalism and career development. Professionalism includes accountability, responsibility, training, knowledge, role modeling, critical thinking, collegiality, team player and ability to influence others. Mentors can assist other healthcare providers in their professional development. Mentoring is part of being a good leader. It is the function of a leader to role model, teach and share what we know with those who follow behind us. They are the future of healthcare, and it is up to us to help them create their own personal path.

 **For your toolkit... Mentoring is part of being a good leader**

Characteristics of Mentoring:

- Coach
- Teach
- Listen
- Provide advice
- Provide situational evaluation
- Make suggestions
- Role play
- Sponsor
- Protect
- Support
- Encourage
- Affirm
- Inspire
- Challenge
- Counsel
- Clarify
- Accept
- Communicate and interrelate
- Kindness
- Patience
- Praise and constructive criticism
- Provides mirror for your views of your self

To navigate challenges in the workplace, as well as do successful career planning, most people find benefits in using a coach or mentor. The old metaphor of climbing the corporate ladder is being replaced by a metaphor that is more about moving out and around different branches of a large tree. Many mid-level managers and healthcare executives are looking at non-traditional paths by which to pursue their career development. These moves can be a lateral move followed by an upward move, then another lateral move.

There is a difference between coaching and mentoring. Mentoring involves a personal relationship that is outside the supervisor-employee relationship. It may last for long periods of time across the span of a career. Mentoring is career-focused and relates to professional development outside a mentee's current span of skills. Mentors provide both personal and professional support. Mentor relationships often cross job boundaries. Mentoring is focused on developing one's career and learning through someone else's expertise. Mentoring relationships include large areas of career development and require a long commitment over time. Mentoring usually creates relationships of value personally and professionally to both the mentee and mentor. (Gates, 2004)

Mentors can be active and passive. Active mentors are those who are willing to coach you as you progress. Passive mentors are role models you can emulate. You need both types in healthcare careers. (See chapter on Career Development)

Mentoring comes with responsibilities on the part of the mentor. There is a commitment to the mentee of time and sharing. You must be caring, knowledgeable and willing to share your own experiences. You need patience and the ability to validate others, while not taking their rejection of your suggestions personally. While many mentors are in leadership positions, it is not necessary to be a manager in order to be an effective mentor. One of my mentors throughout my career has been a diploma program staff nurse.

When you mentor others, you discuss situations and potential challenges. Your role is to listen and advise the mentee. You may write responses for specific requests for information or review certain materials. You meet and network with the mentee, providing sponsorship, introductions and opportunities. Being a mentor allows you to share your knowledge, influence others, role model professional behavior, assist with career development and make a difference by helping someone change their life.

Effective Coaching

While coaching may take place a part of mentoring, executive coaching is usually more formal. Coaching is a process where the coach works with an individual to identify or suggest ways of changing performance to improve results. Coaching usually is focused on developing individuals within their current job or position. The coach and the healthcare provider requesting the coaching usually have a specific agenda or skills to review. This is a different type of coaching than that of life coaching, which is more personal and has become quite popular in the last ten years (2002).

The executive coach assesses the individual's skills and performance, and helps to develop an action plan that will allow the individual to achieve those goals. This is a very structured process and involves advanced complex skills to help the individual expand capacity and take more effective actions. Coaching is usually a short term commitment and may revolve around specific job skills the individual wishes to improve. (Gates, 2004)

Every healthcare employee is capable of being a coach to others who aspire to higher levels of competency and performance. It is part of the professional role to assist others along the learning continuum to increase knowledge and skills competency. Mentoring others is a gift that each of us offers, using experience and wisdom to fully develop talents in the leaders that will follow us.

Effective Precepting

Precepting means showing someone else how to perform your role. A preceptor is selected based on the individuals work skills, knowledge of the unit/department, aptitude for teaching and willingness to participate in orienting new employees. It is helpful to train preceptors how to precept successfully prior to them starting that role. A preceptor is a competent, proficient or expert level (Benner, 2011) healthcare employee with a special area of expertise who is assigned or volunteers to help a novice or advanced beginner level student. The preceptor guides and facilitates the student through the learning activities required to achieve the clinical course objectives. The preceptor actively participates in the evaluation of a student's clinical performance, though the final judgment always rests with the clinical educator for the course.

 **For your toolkit… Precepting means showing someone else how to perform your role. It is a key retention strategy.**

An effective preceptor demonstrates a high level of knowledge, clinical proficiency, professionalism and serves as a clinical instructor to new employees and students in the clinical setting and within numerous healthcare specialties. They also assist with the transition to the clinical environment in order to insure quality patient services, maintains organizational standards, and continuity of patient care in a cost-effective manner.

A preceptor's responsibilities include role model, facilitator, educator, and evaluator. Preceptors may provide input into unit based orientation content and design. They are also encouraged to give input into general orientation design and delivery. Preceptors evaluate the new orientee's performance and participate in planning activities when skill development is indicated. The preceptor only assesses competencies for topics in which s/he has documented competency. Preceptors provide orientee feedback and document the orientee's competencies by using competency checklists.

The educational level and clinical expertise of the preceptor should be greater than the student. Therefore, the education preparation for preceptors of baccalaureate students should be a baccalaureate or higher degree. The minimal clinical experience expected is two years of full-time employment in the special clinical area. This does not have to be two years with a specific organization. The preceptor must have a clear, current, active license in their specialty of practice. The department's director/manager and/or clinical educator must agree to the employee serving as a preceptor.

A preceptor can be identified by the following people: department manager, clinical educator, student, self, school faculty member or another preceptor. Nominations should be in writing, or on the appropriate form for your facility. Preceptor nominations can also be made by verbal communication, such as telephone or written communication, such as e-mail, FAX, letter, or note.

The preceptor functions as a resource person, facilitator, clinical role model, educator, and consultant to the student. The primary role is to provide a learning environment where the student can meet course and individual learning objectives. Preceptors have specific responsibilities. These differ than those of the unit manager or supervisor. Preceptors can work with students and also with new, orienting employees. The responsibilities of the preceptor are to:

- Assist the student/orientee by arranging opportunities and resources to obtain learning experience appropriate to the course and individual learning objectives.

- Assist students in developing learning objectives. This includes advising the student of possible learning opportunities.

- Sign the students individual learning objectives following negotiation for appropriate learning experiences.

- Assist students/orientees in orientation to the facility. This includes philosophy, policies and procedures of the agency and expectations. Examples include dress code, special equipment, emergency situations (fire, disaster, and codes), documentation, charting, medication administration and documentation, specific procedures in your specialty and access to computer system for documentation and retrieval of information, telephone and facsimile use.

- In most situations the student /orientee will need to match the preceptor schedule rather than the other way around. In rare situations, the preceptor may designate another unit staff member to assist the student/ orientee. The designee must be a healthcare professional with sufficient experience to assist the student. The preceptor (or designee) is continuously available when the student/orientee is in the clinical setting.

- Verify student/orientee attendance.

- Provide ongoing evaluation of student/orientee performance to the students and clinical educator.

- Meet with the student midterm and end of term to discuss and document student achievement or lack of achievement of course and individual learning objectives. This is documented on the student learning contract.

- Notify the student and faculty member at any time during the course that a course or individual learning objective is not passed or when a student has not made sufficient progress toward reaching an objective.

- Evaluate the student/orientee's learning, in conjunction with the clinical educator based on the course and individual learning objectives.
- Evaluate the preceptor's own experience for the course

The role of the preceptor is crucial to the success of the new employee or healthcare student. Organization culture must value and support the role by providing a formalized structure for the process. Because students are potential facility employees, every effort should be made to make them feel confident and welcome and to ensure competency. An effective preceptor program using trained experienced preceptors will result in increased healthcare professional retention in health care facilities.

Discussion Questions:
1. Define and explain mentoring.
2. Define and explain coaching.
3. Compare and contrast the differences between coaching and mentoring.
4. Explain the role of preceptor and why it is important to new healthcare workers.

Case Studies:
1. Carol is a middle manager in a community hospital. She noticed a respiratory therapy student crying in the nursing station, with a textbook open next to her. Carol approached the student and asked what was wrong. The student said "I am overwhelmed and I don't understand arterial blood gas values. I am going to fail!" How should Carol handle this student. Why? What should Carol be sure not to do? Why? If this was you as a student, how would you want to be treated?
2. Patricia lectured a lot on healthcare leadership. After a recent conference, an attendee came up to Patricia and asked if Patricia would mentor her. What should Patricia say? Do? How should she follow up?

GENERAL CAREER SKILLS

GENERAL CAREER SKILLS

Chapter Objectives:

1. Define and explain the importance soft skills.
2. List 4 soft skills that are critical to career success
3. Discuss ways to sell your potential with no career experience.
4. Explain the Parieto principle and why it matters in your career.
5. List 5 examples of effective time management.
6. List the 3 keys to managing time.
7. List 3 things your boss wants you to know.
8. Identify and explain the successful communication sequence.
9. List 3 barriers to effective communication.

Key terms

Soft skills   Political skills
Communication   Vibrating poles
Time management   Critical thinking
Parieto principle   What your boss wants
Self-confidence   Management of a meeting
Organizational skills

Important Job Skills

When interviewing for any position, keep in mind that in addition to technical and professional skills, employers are also looking for other skills. These other skills are often called "soft skills" (Vought, 2005). Remember the phrase from your childhood report card "works and plays well with others"? They were talking about a critical soft skill, and there are many more, all of them important for any job in any industry, but particularly in healthcare. There are numerous books and articles about these skills, with different names and labels. Essentially, these are the ones most cited:

- Oral/spoken communication skills
- Written communication skills
- Being truthful and having integrity
- Working effectively with others to accomplish tasks
- Self-motivation/initiative= Doing things without needing to be told or persuaded
- Work ethic/dependability= Being thorough and accurate so others can count on you
- Critical thinking= Challenging things when appropriate and proposing alternatives to consider
- Risk-taking skills= Taking a considered chance on something new, different or unknown
- Flexibility/adaptability= Going with the flow and adjusting with unforeseen circumstances
- Influencing skills= Persuading others to think about or adopt a different point of view
- Organization skills= Being organized and methodical, especially in work-related situations
- Problem-solving skills= Analyzing the potential causes of a problem and creating a solution
- Multicultural skills= Understanding and relating to people who are different from you
- Computer skills= Using basic word-processing, spreadsheet and presentation software as well as the Internet
- Academic/learning skills= Learning new things quickly, thoroughly, and being willing to learn continuously
- Making sure that even the little things are done and done correctly
- Teaching/training skills= Showing other people how to do something in a way that allows them to learn quickly and clearly

- Guiding and supporting others in order to accomplish something
- Relating with other people and communicating with them in everyday interactions
- Handling the stress that accompanies deadlines and other limitations or constraints
- Asking questions in order to learn or clarify something
- Having the imagination to come up with new or out-of-the-box ideas
- Quantitative skills= Compiling and using numbers to study an issue or answer a question
- Research skills= Gathering information to answer questions.
- Time management skills= Using your time wisely and consistently staying on schedule and meeting deadlines. (Vought,2005)

 **For your toolkit....Soft job skills are just as important as clinical competencies**

Selling Yourself with no Experience

One of the biggest challenges in the work place is selling your self without having experience. How do people new to the job market land that first job with little or no real-world work experience? What can you do to jump-start your career if all you have is a brand new diploma and a couple of unrelated summer jobs? Paul Barada believes that what you have to sell is job performance potential, and that's what you need to highlight (2005). Here are some useful tips on how to do just that.

A positive, upbeat, eager, self-confident attitude is critical. However, self-confidence should never be confused with arrogance or smugness. A can-do attitude is fine; that's what you want to radiate during the entire interview process. Demonstrate your willingness to take an entry-level position. Even with a degree, a lack of job experience normally indicates an entry-level position is all you can expect. In fact, an entry-level position is the ideal place to demonstrate your ability to learn quickly, pay your dues and exceed your employer's expectations. Entry-level positions are a great opportunity for you to learn the job. Until you do, you aren't really valuable to an employer. The quicker you can learn the business of your specialty as well as healthcare, the quicker you can expect to move up within the organization.

Demonstrate your desire to learn. Many people fail to make the clear distinction between classroom theory and real-world practice. Realize there is still much you don't know, not just about the job but also the organizational culture, company politics and the day-to-day reality of how things work. Have reasonable salary expectations. Many new job seekers think there's a correlation between industry average salaries and their personal salary expectations. Some job seekers are on a hunt for the job that pays the most money. Because signing bonuses are common for some roles in healthcare, candidates are often weeded out who appear to want to join the company simply for the signing bonus and leave shortly thereafter. Every company is different, and each has different compensation philosophies and policies. Every new employee brings a different set of skills, training, experience and ability to the job.

Be sure to focus on and highlight your soft skills. When employers are asked to rank the three most important skills they look for in new hires, they consistently identify the following: problem solving skills, interpersonal skills and the ability to work effectively with others in a team setting. (Barada, 2005) Make a point to highlight those particular soft skills, including others you have such as leadership, team-building or communication –all of which are transferable from one job to another.

Don't rely on just your degree. Academic credentials are terrific, but they are not all that is needed in the employment setting. A degree is often used to screen job candidates in or out of the prospect pool. The degree signifies the completion of the coursework required. It is usually not an automatic pass into a spectacular first job. Some job seekers see their degree as an entitlement, not as a way to generate opportunities. A degree won't get you a job– it will just open the door.

 **For your toolkit...A degree won't get you a job– it will just open the door.**

With limited work experience, all you really can expect is the chance to prove what you can do. Your job performance potential is the product you have to sell. In return, you can expect the chance to fulfill that potential. To expect more is to invite frustration and failure. Once your career is underway, your past job performance will speak for itself.

What your boss wants you to know

There are certain basic social and political skills that are required in virtually every job. These are the things your boss wishes you knew even if s/he hasn't told you. The survival skills are specific to work settings. If you know them, it is likely one reason you have been successful in your present job so far. In most workplaces, these skills are not spelled out explicitly. Even if you think they are obvious, consider all the people who don't know that~especially your employees.

Come to work. Regularly using all your sick time marks you as an outsider. Everyone is sick once in a while, but regularly missing a day or two here and there, especially on Mondays and Fridays will label you as someone who doesn't have a clue about what it takes to be perceived as productive in your facility.

Identify with your facility. Speak and behave as if what's good for the facility is good for you. Think twice before you complain to other staff members or your boss. If you act as if your boss is your adversary, you are asking for trouble. You are also displaying the perception that your own problems with authority are more important to you than your job.

Watch your boss. Observe how your boss dresses, behaves in meetings, uses her/his time or talks to employees (including you). Learn your boss's priorities and follow them. It doesn't matter if they seem wrong to you. Succeeding at your job often depends on seeing it from your boss's point of view rather than your own. If you have a boss that displays behaviors that you see are perceived as unacceptable by fellow employees or administrators, take note of that as well. You can always learn what *not* to do at the same time you are learning what to do well.

Have a professional appearance. Every facility has its own standards for dress and a dress code. It is best to conform to it. A rule of thumb for dressing at work if you do not need to meet specific clinical care standards is to not wear anything that will call attention to you. Following the dress code does not mean you can't have your own style. Using your style within the confines of the dress standards will identify you as both conforming and creative.

Be pleasant. Make an effort to get along with folks you work with. If you are upset with someone, try and deal calmly, courteously and directly with that person. Don't take your problems to everyone you interact with. Eliminate eye ball rolling and big frowns. Do your best to avoid participating in squabbles with co-workers– it will ruin your professional image.

Take direction and criticism. It would be great if your boss were more specific and positive with her/his feedback. But, work is just like poker. You need to play the hand you're dealt.

Do your job as if it were worth doing. Make it a point to learn all you can about your job and what it involves. Give your best effort to all parts of your job. It's a bad idea to make your boss remind you about the things you are not doing well.

Have a sense of humor. No one likes to work with people who take themselves too seriously. Keep a sense of humor about your politics, illnesses, pets and children.

Let go of vibrating poles. There are multiple issues in healthcare organizations that can make you crazy. Our natural tendency is to try and control things so we can "fix" them. Many healthcare facilities are extremely dysfunctional, so we can't change anything. As we continue to try and control whatever is dysfunctional, the more frustrated we get, and still nothing changes. A healthcare organization is the equivalent of a vibrating pole. The temptation is to hang on to the pole to make it stop vibrating. In reality, that makes both you and the pole vibrate. The answer is to let go of the pole. Not easy to do in work settings, but the only thing that will save your sanity.

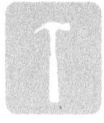 **For your toolkit...Survival advice from your Boss**

- **Come to work**
- **Identify with your facility**
- **Watch your boss to identify priorities**
- **Look professional**
- **Be pleasant**
- **Take direction and criticism gracefully**
- **Do your job well**
- **Have a sense of humor**
- **Let go of vibrating poles**

 ## Turner Employee Survival Skills List©

- Come to work
- Don't badmouth your organization
- Watch your boss for clues, pet peeves, needs and expectations
- Provide your boss what s/he needs, not what you think s/he should have
- Be professional
- Be kind and pleasant
- Have a sense of humor
- Be willing to take direction and criticism
- Do your work in a way that shows you care about your job
- Let go of vibrating poles

Turner Healthcare © 2004

TIME MANAGEMENT

"The past is gone-the future may never be and all we have of the present is an invisible instant that is gone before we can say it is here."

Even if you are not a manager, everyone can use ideas and tools to better manage time. More effective management of your time can mean that you have more time in your personal life to do the things you enjoy. These organizing skills will give you better time management as well as methods to better organize your energy and resources.

Time management is not about the amount of time we have. It is how we utilize the time that is available to us. Most people believe they do not have control over their time. When consistently applied, time management skills will assist you in maximizing your tine to achieve your personal and professional goals. Time is without a doubt our most valuable resource. Yet in spite of its preciousness, there is hardly anything else that we squander so thoughtlessly.

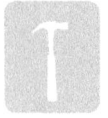 **For your toolkit... Time management is not about the amount of time we have. It is how we utilize the time that is available to us.**

Time has special characteristics. You can't accelerate its speed nor can you slow it down. You can't store it or recover time you have lost. Time is a gift that you cannot buy or sell. It cannot be controlled. Time simply slips away endlessly and relentlessly 1440 minutes every day no mater who you are or what you do with your time. Because of these unique characteristics, one of the measures of success is determined by how well s/he manages or invests time. Time management is an individual activity, and the staff members who manage their time well are usually the best.

There are many reasons why people don't manage their work time well. Consider the ones that apply to you:

I don't manage my time well because:

- There are too many uncontrollable interruptions
- I am a pressure worker who produces best when faced with short time schedules

- I delay things I don't like to do
- I don't plan; I react
- I am usually too tired and have too little time to think about how I should spend my time
- I am too preoccupied
- I don't like my job
- I have health problems
- I am a perfectionist and never plan for enough time for a project
- I have too many chance meetings in the halls
- I don't know how to manage my time
- Others don't manage their time well and impose on me
- I have too many demands
- Managing my time is boring and too mechanistic
- I can't prioritize because everything seems important
- Time management is not possible
- I don't delegate well
- I am a procrastinator
- I manage by crisis
- I don't have adequate support activities
- I have to attend too many meetings
- There is too little communication
- I am often confused about tasks I should do
- I don't have any goals

These barriers and excuses keep you from managing your time effectively. You don't practice time management when you have more time. You have more time when you practice time management. You can't change the way you have managed your time in the past, but you can manage your present opportunities and plan for the future.

Healthcare staff and managers must focus on their daily priorities to enable them to reach their overall objectives. They must constantly organize themselves and their time. Effective time management skills for both staff and managers include:

- Develop objectives and priorities
- Analyze how you use your time
- Have a results-oriented plan (outcomes-based)
- Organize for achievement
- Control unproductive deviations or time wasters

Follow-up with periodic reviews to see how effectively you have used your time.

Peter Drucker, a well known management consultant and writer, believes that the key to effectiveness is to know where our time should be spent for the results we want. (2010) The Pareto Principle (80/20) provides that 80% of our results come from 20% of what we do. Therefore, it appears that we tend to spend a lot of our time on low value activities. This means that we are not utilizing our time for the maximum outcomes or results.

When evaluating your current time management approach, you need to consider these questions about what you do:

- Does it relate to my job objectives?
- What is the immediacy of what I am doing?
- Why am I doing it? Could others do it?
- Is the time I spend proportionately matched to the priorities of my responsibilities?

Make a list of the ten most common things you do in your job. Out of those ten listed activities, check the two items that yield 80% of your results and objectives. What priorities do these activities have in your day? Do you focus on them or do you just fit them in when you can? It is important to review how your actual work flow may be getting in your way of accomplishing your objectives. We all have the same amount of time; the difference is how we use it. Time is a constant factor. It's what you do with the time that matters. The key to excellence is self-management, not time management.

There are some people who get everything done. It is easy to assume that you will be needed more if you don't get everything done. This is a myth. Another myth is to think that you can do more than one thing at a time. While multi-tasking is commonplace, it is tough to do more than one thing at a time and do it effectively. The biggest misconception about time management is that waiting for a crisis is a good way to prioritize. While waiting until a crisis certainly creates lots of motivation (and possibly fear), good planning eliminates the need for putting out fires. Being proactive causes you less work in the end because you avert the problems and time consuming clean up jobs.

Other challenges are those individuals who are procrastinators or perfectionists. Many people are both. Those juggling dozens of daily tasks and desires will not get things done if they use the "if something's worth doing, its' worth doing well." Actually, those who apply extreme perfectionism standards to almost everything they do are almost always underachievers. That is because they tend to take too much time on unimportant tasks and lose momentum for the really important things. Successful healthcare staff knows how to apply a flexible standard to each task depending on its value. When appropriate, they are not above doing a "quick and dirty" job. An example of this strategy would be scanning a professional journal instead of reading it word for word. The "quick and dirty" strategy usually relates to non-clinical tasks. Don't use this method when carrying out clinical patient procedures.

There are many things that are time wasters. They limit your effectiveness. You can form new habits for each time waster. Evaluate these time wasters and see which ones get in your way of managing your goals and priorities:
- Attending meetings that don't matter
- Procrastinating often
- Too many phone conversations
- Drop in visitors that interrupt you
- No specific plan for the day
- No specific and measurable business goals
- Spend most of your time on routine tasks and trivia
- Your desk/work area is cluttered
- Being indecisive

- Routinely have afternoon drowsiness
- You have to repeat instructions /directions to subordinates
- Paperwork takes up a huge part of your day
- You try and do it all to be successful
- Unexpected problems cause you to react and divert other priorities
- You routinely join the "coffee break" folks?
- You lack specific time blocks to work on priorities

Any of the above items that you recognize as your own behavior are limiting your effectiveness. Pick one area and minimize its effect as a time waster.

There are ways to gain time. You can incorporate them into your daily lives to enable you to better accomplish your personal and professional goals. Each one you implement will help you gain time:

- *Meetings:* Only hold meetings with an agenda. Start on time, be on tie and end on time. Delegate any meetings you can to others. Schedule meetings back to back

- *Procrastination:* Set deadlines and specific priorities. Promise results in writing to another person. Break large projects into small ones.

- *Phone interruptions:* when working on top projects/issues, have calls screened or let voicemail pick it up. Get out of your office. Limit time of routine phone contacts.

- *Drop in visitors:* Stand and talk to the visitor. Explain that you would love to talk but cannot do so now. Be direct but polite. Close your door when you are working.

- *Daily plan:* Use one that is simple. Every day, write down six things to do, in order of priority. Start with item 1 and work one at a time. Don't worry if you don't finish all the items. Transfer the unfinished items to the next day's list.

- *Goals:* Set business and personal goals. It works to help make you more productive. Lack of direction wastes time and efforts. Goal setting is one of the greatest success secrets of all time.

- *Routine and trivia:* Do routine or trivial things by schedule. Don't do it whenever it pops up. Save junk mail, phone calls or reading for times you have lower energy or non prime time.

- *Cluttered desk:* Clean off your desk, put anything you can out of sight so you are not distracted. Do one priority at a time. Consider creating a minimal number of papers to have on your desk that represent priorities, e.g. three or four.

- *Indecision:* Gather information and act. Take calculated risks, which is a manager's job. Keep others appropriately involved or informed of your decisions.

- *Directions:* Be specific and if you need to, ask subordinates to paraphrase or repeat your instructions back to you. Always follow up to check results and consider putting detailed or complex instructions in writing.

- *Paperwork:* Call, don't write memos whenever possible. Handle mail only once. Write notes on letters/memos and return them instead of doing another separate letter or memo. Any time you pick up a piece of paper, do something with it, including filing or throwing it away. Don't stack it up to "do something with later." I stand at the recycle bin and sort mail. Anything that is junk mail goes directly into the recycler and never comes into the house.

- *Afternoon drowsiness:* Take a walk at noon or work out in a health club. Eat a light lunch. Consider a short walk or high protein snack in the afternoon to counteract the drowsiness. Don't eat high carbohydrate or high sugar foods at lunch or for a snack.

- *Trying to do it all:* Focus on the 20% of your tasks that yield 80% of your results. Delegate to others whenever possible. Say no sometimes. Give yourself a break occasionally. You will end up being more effective.

- *Unexpected problems:* Handle them swiftly if they are urgent. Don't fret or worry about what you have done. You can't be a prophet and plan for everything. Make sure you train and empower your staff to solve their own problems when they can. Ask "what are you going to do? " Don't accept the problem for fixing if the staff members can solve it on their own.

- *Coffee klatsches:* If you are committed to excellence and getting your job done, skip the coffee breaks. Be social at a different time. This is not the same as "management by walking around," discussed in the supervision/management chapter

71

- *Interruptions:* When working on priorities, have your phone calls screened. Close your door or work in a different location. Establish quiet hours and get things done during the day. You don't have to work longer hours to be effective.

There are several ways to gain time. Real time management is self management. You can't manage time, but you can manage yourself. Time is constant, 168 hours per week. What you do with those hours is the secret to getting more done. One of the most efficient physicians I know says "we all have the same twenty-four hours; I just choose to do more with mine." To manage yourself better, you must be willing to change. New habits must replace old habits. Change is usually uncomfortable at first. With persistence and repetition, this can be overcome. The key to self-management is to manage your response to an event. Good time managers are good at controlling their responses to events they can't control. Use the time gaining techniques. How you respond to time wasters depends on your attitude and your willingness to plan.

You can create your own time analysis and develop a personal self management program. Outline the objectives you want to accomplish this week. Prioritize those objectives according to their importance to you. Make sure you take some time out at the beginning or end of the day (for the next day) to do your daily to do list. Review yesterday's list and do the next day's list. Make sure to highlight the tasks you must complete today. The time of day you plan depends on when you are most alert and have some quiet time to concentrate and reflect.

Be prepared for your to do list strategy to be sabotaged and for things to get in the way. You should always plan on "Murphy's law" being in effect. This law is "whatever can go wrong, will go wrong." The other given is that everything always takes longer than you think. Keep in mind there are 3 keys to managing time.

1. Assess time by determining if objectives are realistic in the allotted time you made.
2. Set priorities so that what is important is what is accomplished.
3. Stick to your plan and be single-minded. Eliminate your time wasting habits.

If you are an effective supervisor, you know the abilities, initiatives and dependability of each subordinate. Then delegate accordingly. Reduce the routine order of things and schedule similar tasks together whenever possible. Additional ideas for helping yourself become better organized include:

- De-clutter your desk each day so you are not losing documents and getting distracted.

- Consolidate similar tasks

- Before making a call or visit, outline the basic points to be covered. On the telephone, identify yourself immediately and spend minimal time on chit chat. If a personal visit is necessary, make an appointment first.

- Delegate what is appropriate. Develop your subordinates to assume routine tasks, plan and think creatively and to handle more responsibility to free you up to do more supervisory tasks.

- Plan concentrated time blocks for those projects and problems that need analysis and uninterrupted time. When you are interrupted, you often have to go back over material you covered before the interruption. Schedule a time to make and return phone calls.

- Avoid procrastination and work on priority items to complete them

- Practice clear and direct communication. Unclear directions and communication wastes yours and others time by causing things to be redone and re-explained.

- Practice streamlined reading by finding central thoughts, major themes, skimming materials. Read whole thoughts and phrases at a time to improve speed and comprehension.

- Sort your papers on your desk by using:

  i. *Toss*– if the paper has no value, don't keep it. Throw it away now and don't keep it to throw away later.

  ii. *Refer*– pass papers onto subordinates or appropriate coworkers when possible. Write a note on the document to the person you are sending it to. Put it in the out box.

  iii. *Act*– a paper requiring a response from you should be put in an action file.

    iv. *File*—a paper that might have future value for you should be placed in a desk/cabinet file. If your file cabinets are a distance from your desk, stack all items to be filed together, and take them at one time to the cabinet.

    v. Schedule a time each day to process/sort mail and answer it

    vi. Keep track of complex, deferred and referred actions with a calendar or index cards in a "holding status" file.

    vii. Make a quick desk check at the end of each day to be sure all papers have been sorted as above.

- Plan meetings carefully. They are good for generating ideas, sharing information, and making decisions that require group input.

- Call a meeting if you need to:
  - i. Define goals
  - ii. Reach group judgments on decisions
  - iii. Discover, analyze or solve a problem
  - iv. Gain acceptance for an idea, program, decision or change
  - v. Reconcile conflicting view
  - vi. Provide essential information
  - vii. Assure understanding of policy, methods or decisions
  - viii. Obtain immediate reactions when speedy responses to a problem

- *DO NOT* use a meeting format if you:
  - o Can communicate in other medium, such as telephone, memo, email and get results
  - o There is insufficient time for adequate preparation
  - o One or more key participants are not available
  - o Time is not convenient
  - o Net return isn't realized in view of cost of meeting

- Make sure when you call a meeting that you:
  - o Prepare for the meeting
  - o Start and end on time (!)

- ○ Get to the point
- ○ Watch group dynamics. Are people frustrated? Angry? Contributing? Complaining about wasting time?
- ○ Summarize accomplishments
- ○ Follow-up with minutes and action items.
- ○ Keep tabs on action item progress

Keep in mind as you try all these new techniques that it takes a minimum of twenty one days to reinforce positive changes in behavior. Remember the rewards to effective tie management will work in both your professional and personal life and last a lifetime. Successful staff and managers have control of their time because they are organized for achievement.

Evaluate your Communication Styles-It Does Affect your Career

There are numerous definitions for communication. It is an active process, not a static one. Communication is the sending and receiving of information, feelings and attitudes, both verbally and non-verbally, that produces a response (2012). In effective communication, a message is transmitted and received, but the real process of communicating starts when the receiver provides a response to the sender.

Effective communication occurs between two persons when the receiver interprets the sender's message the same way that the sender intended it. Both the sender and the receiver are affected by his/her personal background, attitudes, perceptions, emotions, opinions, education and experience. There is a specific meaning in the message the sender intends to send. There are also symbols used to communicate-both verbally and non-verbally. The message essentially has no meaning until it is actually received by the receiver. The receiver is also affected by personal background, attitudes, perceptions, emotions, opinions, education and experience. (Turner, 1999) A successful communication sequence looks like this:

Sender→ Meaning→ Message→ Symbols→ Meaning→ Receiver (Turner, 1999)

Essentially, this means that the same factors that create effective communication can also be barriers to effective communications. For example, a speaker's ethnic background can make that person great at communicating with other members of the same ethnicity; however, the speaker may not be equally as effective when speaking to an ethnically diverse audience (Turner, 1999)

Elements of Communication:

- Sender
- Receiver
- Message (meaning the sender wants to send)
- Symbols (how the message is sent e.g. verbal, non verbal)
- Message (the meaning actually received)

Other barriers to effective communication include:

- Preconceived assumptions and stereotypes
- Distractions like extraneous noise, too many people talking at once
- Emotional triggers like judgmental statements or expression of feelings that create listener resentment and defensiveness e.g. "What did you do now?"
- Confusing or complex language that has a different meaning to sender and receiver e.g. "Did the patient void?"
- Physical barriers e.g. hearing impairment
- Being unprepared
- Failure to be direct and concise
- Feelings of intimidation in a high-pressure environment
- Poor timing because the receiver is unable or not ready to listen. (Turner, 1998)

Being insensitive can also damage communication y causing the sender or receiver to look at the situation from only one point of view. Non verbal gestures, movements such as tapping, avoiding eye contact, voice tone, pitch , inflection and mumbling also cause ineffective communication.

Healthcare staff can use strategies to improve communication and become successful at communication in the workplace. During stressful times, effective communication becomes critical. Because many staff are often overwhelmed and frustrated, these strategies become even more important. Try using an open-ended style of questioning. Open-ended questions are questions requiring more than a yes or now answer. Select the proper environment to have your conversation. Offering criticism to a co-worker at a nurses' station is not only rude, but unkind. Privacy is an important consideration for staff members and patients, as well as anyone involved in a conflict or stress producing situation.

Timing of communication is crucial. It may not be a good idea to bring up a conflict to your boss on a bad day or on his/her birthday. Be selective when choosing to discuss conflicts. Send your own message by using first-person singular pronouns and explanations. "I feel...." This type of personal ownership includes clearly taking responsibility for the ideas and feelings that one expresses. People disown their messages when they use phrases like "most people" or "our group." This type of language makes it difficult for listeners to tell whether the individuals really think and feel what they are saying or whether they are repeating thoughts and feelings of others.

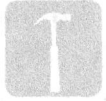 **For your toolkit... Your timing of communication is crucial.**

Ask for feedback on how your messages are received. To communicate effectively, you must be aware of how the receiver is interpreting and processing your messages. The only way to be sure is to continually seek feedback as to what meanings the receiver is attaching to your messages. Make the message appropriate to the receiver's frame of reference. Use different appropriate words and depths of explanation for an expert in the field, and a novice, a child and an adult, your boss and a co-worker.

Non-verbal communication is the most important aspect of communication and often the most ignored. Body language is 55% of communication. Tone of voice is 38%. The actual words stated comprise only 7%of the communicated message. (2012) Maintaining good eye contact instills credibility and honesty in the receiver. Make verbal and non-verbal messages consistent and congruent. Every face to face communication involves both verbal and non verbal messages. Usually these messages are congruent. Problems arise when a person's verbal and non verbal messages are contradictory because the non verbal messages do not support the verbal message and the receiver is confused.

Make your messages compete and specific. Include clear statements of necessary information the receiver needs in order to comprehend the message. Being complete and specific seems obvious, but often people do no communicate the frame of reference they are using, the assumptions they are making, the intentions they have in communicating, or the leaps in thinking they are making.

Focus on issues and behaviors, not people. Describe others' behavior without evaluating or interpreting. When reacting to the behavior or others, be sure to describe their behavior e.g. "you keep interrupting me" rather than evaluating it, e.g. you're a rotten self-centered egotist who won't listen to anyone else's ideas." Get rid of "excess baggage" by concentrating on just the basic communication experience you are involved in. Learn to minimize redundancy, excessive detail, irrelevant information, and distractions. Outline in your mind what you way to say.

Listening is a critical element of the communication process. Listening skills can be developed. Anyone who wants to get the most out off a dialogue must be both a good speaker and a good listener. Types of listening are defined as passive and active. Passive listening is listening that you don't have to work at, such as to TV and music. Active listening requires full attention in order to hear and understand the entire message.

For your toolkit... Listening is critical to your success.

To be successful at active listening, you must listen for the purpose of understanding what is meant, not for the purpose of readying yourself for a reply(!) Try to listen to the whole message first: don't interpret too quickly what the speaker is trying to say. Attempt to put aside your own views and opinions while actively listening. Put yourself in the speaker's shoes, and try to understand how s/he views the world.

Try to keep your thoughts from being interrupted by how you plan to respond. Don't trust your intuition. Validate the message with the sender. Expect the speaker to use different words than you might and try not to make snap judgments about what you are hearing. There are different styles of communication that work in different situations. It is important for healthcare staff to be familiar with and competent in all these types of communication.

Discussion Questions:

1. Discuss and explain the importance soft skills.
2. Identify 4 soft skills that are critical to career success and why.
3. Discuss ways to sell your potential with no career experience.
4. Explain the Parieto principle and why it matters in your career.
5. Discuss and identify effective time management skills.
6. Discuss the keys to managing time and how to use them.
7. Discuss and explain the concept of "things your boss wants you to know". List examples.
8. Discuss and explain the successful communication sequence.
9. Discuss barriers to effective communication, and why they happen.

Case Studies:

1. Eileen is new in her role as CEO of a hospital non-profit foundation (fund raising arm). Her role is to manage existing donations as well as obtain more monies. She is also in charge of the operations of a six person department. She reports to the facility CEO and sits on the management council. What skills are most important in her role? Why?

2. Rita is an Emergency Department (ED) nurse who applied for a new role as Pre-Hospital Care coordinator. It is a promotion within the ED. When she was not selected, she wrote a letter to the Department manager, the VP of Patient Care, the Chief of the Medical Staff and the hospital CEO. Why do you think she did this? Was this appropriate? Why or why not? What could she have done differently?

HEALTHCARE ROLES

"Be the change that you want to see in the world."
-Mahatma Gandhi

HEALTHCARE ROLES

Chapter Objectives:

1. Identify 5 non-clinical roles available in hospitals, and the additional education required, if any, for each role.
2. List 3 non-clinical roles outside hospitals.
3. Explain concept of advanced practice nursing and give examples of roles.
4. Identify 3 advanced practice roles for other healthcare specialties and explain each.

Key terms

Non clinical role   Healthcare executive roles
Advanced practice role   Special focused roles
Community based roles   Occupational Outlook Handbook

Non Clinical Roles in Hospitals

What can you do besides clinical healthcare in a hospital?

When providing direct patient loses its appeal, you can renew your energy by working in a non-clinical specialty. You can draw on your clinical experience and still love healthcare. There are numerous jobs available for experienced healthcare workers who are no longer able or willing to deliver bedside or direct clinical care. These jobs are few and far between, but most healthcare facilities have them. They are healthcare specialty roles. Some are administrative, others are considered middle management or senior executive positions.

Patient/Staff Educators

Clinical healthcare worker educators help patients and their families understand the patient's condition prior to discharge, and what to do for the patient once they are all at home. Educators offer independent classes and they can also work in outpatient areas like cardiac rehabilitation, diabetes education or childbirth preparation. In most facilities, clinical educators also orient and train new healthcare workers and provide additional courses and in-service training for staff healthcare workers. Clinical healthcare worker educators possess at least a bachelor's degree and many are nurses. However, you do not have to be a nurse to be a clinical educator. Some have advanced clinical training in a specialty, and others are professional healthcare educators.

While they must be able to communicate clearly, healthcare educators must enjoy teaching. A passionate educator will get students excited about the subject as well. Healthcare educators need to be able to write education plans, organize courses, and have excellent time management, written and oral communication skills.

Quality Improvement

Healthcare workers involved in quality improvement constantly ask the question of "how can this be improved or done better?" Healthcare workers in this role review a healthcare institution's methods and processes. Their work is evidence-based and outcome-focused. By studying patient populations, they analyze systems to determine how to correct problems and improve quality of care. In short, they strive to prevent future problems by studying past mistakes (Mehallow, 2005).

Healthcare workers in this role usually have a bachelor's degree in a healthcare field. Many are registered nurses, but it is not mandatory. Being a certified professional in healthcare quality (CPHQ) is a definite plus, but not all employers require that certification. The Healthcare Quality Certification Board oversees CPHQ testing. In most facilities, healthcare workers involved in quality improvement work in a department outside of patient care that reports to a senior executive. Excellent written and oral communication skills are a must, along with political savvy and patience.

Risk Managers

Risk management is closely tied to quality improvement. Risk managers also search for the root causes of mistakes to help improve systems and processes. Healthcare workers are great in this role because they are already thinking about patients using the patient care process. Job opportunities for risk managers are increasing at hospitals, and all types of clinical settings. Even insurance companies and law practices use healthcare workers in these roles. Risk-management healthcare workers review patient records before and after lawsuits are filed and during legal proceedings. Risk managers work with senior medical and administrative staff. These jobs require patience, tact and political savvy plus excellent communication, conflict resolution and writing skills.

Most risk-management healthcare workers hold at least a bachelor's degree and risk-management certification, which is available from the American Hospital Association Certification Center, the American Board of Quality Assurance and Utilization Review Physicians and some colleges.

Case Managers

Case managers are the choreographers of the patient care experience. They coordinate all the health care team members, ensuring continuity and that everyone understands what is happening with the patients. As hospitals discharge patients more quickly and managed-care organizations increasingly oversee patient care, the need for case managers has increased. The aging population is generating more opportunities in long-term care and home healthcare as well (Mehallow, 2005).

The demand for healthcare case managers is increasing and more facilities are looking for healthcare workers who have both strong clinical experience and certification in case management. Many case managers are nurses, but again, it is not usually required. The two primary certifying bodies are the Commission for Case Manager Certification and the American Healthcare workers Credentialing Center. Case managers are expected to achieve the highest achievable patient outcome with the shortest possible hospitalization. This role requires healthcare workers who are self-directed, proactive and able to create change. Characteristics needed to be successful in this role include patience, diplomacy and politically astuteness.

Chart Auditors:

Healthcare workers often serve as financial chart auditors in their specialty. The role requires review of patient charts after discharge to ensure appropriate documentation for proper billing and coding. There are also chart auditors that work in quality management and review charts for appropriate clinical documentation of all aspects of patient care, including healthcare workers. Many chart auditors are diploma or associate degree healthcare graduates. A graduate degree is not required by most facilities for this role. Chart auditors need excellent reading skills and the ability to communicate their findings to others. Political savvy is a plus, as folks in this role must ask other clinicians to improve or revise their chart documentation.

Patient Advocates

Healthcare workers can also serve as patient advocate. This role is customer-service focused and primarily patient advocates handle patient complaints. This is an excellent role for a healthcare worker with a physical disability that limits the active tasks of bedside health care, or a mature healthcare worker who can no longer tolerate the physical demands of bedside healthcare. No additional education or training is required for this role. Patient advocates need excellent listening skills, patience and a solution-focused problem solving perspective.

Preceptors

More and more hospitals are creating formal positions for experienced healthcare workers to guide new healthcare workers through that critical first year on the job. As hospitals recognize the connection between strong preceptor skills and new grad retention rates, more formalized programs for training preceptors are being developed. Preceptors are experienced healthcare workers who enjoy teaching and working with new healthcare workers and new graduates. Patience is a must, plus a positive attitude and ability to make people feel comfortable asking questions. No additional formal healthcare education is required for this role, although many hospitals require formal preceptor training before doing this type of work. This is a great role for an older healthcare worker no longer able to perform bedside healthcare.

Clinical Information System Consultants

Many healthcare facilities are looking towards healthcare workers to assist in converting existing patient data processes to electronic medical record systems. Healthcare workers' clinical knowledge and ability to understand all the steps in a patient hospitalization make them the perfect project coordinator. These roles require patience, technology knowledge and the ability to work between the healthcare workers and information technology worlds. Political savvy is a plus, because in this role you will function as a change agent and project champion. Additional education and training is usually not required.

Your primary healthcare education and clinical experience provide lots of options once you determine that bedside healthcare is no longer a viable career option. To assess these types of jobs, ask to job shadow with someone currently in the role to see if it is a fit for you.

Clinical Informatics Specialists

The hospital implementation of information technology has given healthcare workers added responsibility throughout the country. However, it has also provided new professional specialties. Clinical informatics is one of them. These healthcare workers are part of a clinical team that promotes patient care through the design, implementation, and maintenance of the hospital's clinical information system. (DeRitis, 2004) Clinical systems usually interface with other hospital systems, like the pharmacy, ER, laboratory and registration systems. These interfaces support clinical decision making and are critical to patient care issues.

Healthcare workers can fill these roles and assist with development of these systems. Their clinical mentality becomes crucial in designing the finished product. Technology is also advancing at the bedside, with many facilities implementing personal PDAs for healthcare workers documentation. Bar coding patient admission armbands and medications are other bedside advancements that clinical informatics specialists are involved in.

HEALTHCARE ROLES OUTSIDE THE HOSPITAL

Healthcare workers Roles in the Community

Mid-career healthcare workers can reinvent themselves without starting over. Experienced healthcare workers can apply their clinical skills and experience outside of the hospital. Take a look at these career possibilities. One of them may allow you to realign or rediscover your passion for healthcare workers.

Correctional Healthcare workers

There are two million inmates and juvenile offenders behind bars in this country. Healthcare workers who work with them deal with a range of medical problems, from toothaches to trauma. Most inmates do not have easy access to healthcare. Correctional healthcare workers enjoy taking care of people who need a lot of services and education. The biggest challenge of correctional healthcare workers is the ability to look at a person not by what they do, but for who they are. This is not a role for everyone, but those who do it, love it. Correctional healthcare workers work autonomously. They assess new inmates, manage the chronic diseases and mental illnesses of long-term prisoners and respond to acute illnesses and injuries. Inmates as a population have more complex and acute healthcare needs than the general community population. These healthcare workers must be confident, mature and well-rounded.

Healthcare workers in prisons and jails are as safe as in the community, because correctional officers are always nearby and the environments are carefully controlled. No additional educational credentials are required, but training on how to work in a correctional setting is provided on the job. Patience, excellent communication skills and a non-judgmental attitude are musts for this role.

Forensic Healthcare workers

Healthcare workers have always worked with victims and perpetrators of violent crime, but it wasn't until the early 'nineties that "forensic healthcare workers" became a common description for this work. Now, there are almost 8000 registered healthcare workers (many but not all are RNs) who regularly fill forensic-healthcare roles. Some work full-time investigating deaths or treating violent offenders at psychiatric facilities and others moonlight as Sexual Assault Healthcare worker Examiners (SANE) or legal healthcare worker consultants (Mehallow, 2005).

Hollywood's portrayal of forensic healthcare workers in shows such as CSI is misleading. Forensic healthcare workers must be patient, methodical and thorough in assessments in order to withstand the scrutiny of court. Healthcare workers assess crime victims and perpetrators to look for even the smallest sign of injury to show whether an assault did or did not occur. Additional specialty training is required for this role. Healthcare workers who are interested in this specialty field can get a taste of forensic healthcare workers by participating in one of the 400 SANE training programs offered at hospitals and other sites around the country (Mehallow, 2005).

Holistic Healthcare workers

Holistic healthcare workers are a growing specialty. Healthcare consumers' acceptance of the philosophy that treating the whole person is better than treating just a disease or symptom has caused this field to expand exponentially in the last decade. Improved insurance coverage for alternative healthcare practices has also allowed more patients to explore this care option. Any healthcare worker who embraces the mind/body/spirit connection and empowers patients to participate in their own healing practices holism.

In addition to embracing the holistic philosophy, many healthcare workers become proficient and earn certification or licensure in other healing modalities as therapeutic massage, aromatherapy, imagery, acupuncture, herbology or Reiki. These practices complement Western medicine, and are frequently encouraged by traditional physicians. While some practitioners work full-time healthcare jobs and practice their healing modality on the side, others take positions in holistic wellness centers, spas, health clubs and physicians' offices. Additional education is required to practice in this specialty (Mehallow, 2005)

Parish Healthcare workers

The most important role of a parish healthcare worker is helping people understand how faith and health work together. Parish healthcare workers promote healthful living by educating and counseling parishioners on exercise and nutrition, advocating for community health, helping sick parishioners navigate the medical system, and developing support groups for bereavement, parenting, divorce and other issues. Many of these roles are held by RNs, but it is not a requirement. There has been a recent expansion in parish healthcare in some parts of the US, led by expansive health/wellness programs at specific congregations, such as the Daniel Plan, offered by Saddleback Community Church in Lake Forest, California.

Many parish healthcare worker roles are unpaid. The paid ones usually work 20 hours or less per week. Healthcare workers interested in this specialty should work with their own churches to get started or investigate whether any local hospitals sponsor parish healthcare worker outreach programs. There is usually no additional training required for this specialty. Many retired healthcare workers seek these roles to continue healthcare workers while serving the community (Mehallow, 2005).

Legal Healthcare Consulting

Legal healthcare worker consultants work at the cross over between medicine and law, consulting with attorneys and others in the legal arena on medical malpractice, personal injury, workers' compensation and other healthcare-related cases. The legal healthcare consultant's main function is educating attorneys, and these healthcare workers are a huge asset to them. Many legal healthcare consultants work on staff at law firms, insurance companies and other institutions. Others work independently, charging an hourly fee for their work. Legal healthcare worker consulting allows healthcare workers to branch out of the clinical setting while still making use of their experience and knowledge. Functions of a legal healthcare consultant include interviewing clients, reviewing medical records, researching and summarizing medical literature, assisting with evaluation of liabilities and damages, assisting with depositions, preparing exhibits, and working with expert witnesses.

Independent legal healthcare consultants perform many of the same tasks as their in-house counterparts. In addition, they sometimes serve as expert witnesses at depositions or trials, where they are called upon to testify about whether healthcare workers care deviated from established standards of care. Many independent legal healthcare consultants, including still work full- or part-time in the hospital. The demand is higher for independent legal healthcare consultants who are currently working in the field and can offer the most informed opinions on healthcare issues.

The field of legal healthcare consulting has grown tremendously and there are now thousands of legal healthcare consultants in practice across the nation. The only prerequisite to becoming a legal healthcare consultant is clinical experience in your specialty. Many are RNs, but that is not a requirement. While formal training in legal healthcare worker consulting is not required to practice, training and educational programs are available at universities, community colleges, nonprofits and for-profit organizations.

Healthcare Consultant

Does it sound exciting to strike out on your own? Many healthcare workers carve out lucrative niches as consultants, offering data analysis, strategic planning, project management or architectural services. Besides health and methodology expertise, consultants must have the ability to communicate in a way that the client understands. Healthcare workers need to understand and have a feel for the client's content area. You must be able to market and sell your services. That includes managing relationships, negotiating and closing a deal, estimating jobs accurately and figuring out market-rate pricing.

Consultants need to identify a broad area that they can specialize in. Failing to be too specific at what you can consult on limits your credibility, but not being broad enough allow you to be pigeon-holed into only consulting about certain things. You must also build an alternative source of income for six months to one year, as it takes that long to generate clients and a consistent revenue stream. Keep in mind that often there is a time lag between getting a referral and actually starting the work. You need to have a plan for income and work in the middle of the time lag.

Medical Office Manager

Healthcare workers are well-suited to running a physician's office, a hectic job requiring a wide range of skills and constant multitasking. HIPAA, OSHA and compliance laws make this position much more complex than in the past. Office managers must understand billing and coding as well as clinical care issues. This is a great role for a healthcare worker no longer able to handle the physical aspects of bedside healthcare workers.

The Professional Association of Health Care Office Management, the Practice Management Institute and the Association of Registered Health Care Professionals offer certification programs for office managers. While most office managers learned on the job, some community colleges now offer associate's degrees in healthcare office management. (Mehallow, 2005)

Research Healthcare worker

Research healthcare workers are the eyes, ears and hands that conduct much of today's clinical research. Staff research healthcare workers participate in clinical trials that evaluate new drugs and medical devices. They work with the principal investigator and research coordinators. They evaluate potential studies, screen and schedule patients, coordinate patient visits according to protocols, review patient progress and help report study results. Research healthcare workers can also conduct research related to the practice of healthcare. They may evaluate and study healthcare practices, procedures or care philosophies with the sole purpose of improving healthcare practice.

Research healthcare workers typically work in academic medical centers, educational institutions, pharmaceutical companies and private research foundations, but private-practice physicians are now also hiring research healthcare workers. Most research positions require a master's prepared healthcare worker. (Mehallow, 2005)

Case Managers

Distinct from hospital case managers who coordinate patient care, these professionals work for managed-care companies, home-care agencies, healthcare workers agencies and management-services organizations to minimize duplication of care and services and maximize clinical and financial outcomes.

These healthcare workers must understand Medicare/Medicaid regulations, managed-care guidelines and the care guidelines issued by the Joint Commission on Accreditation of Healthcare Organizations. Case managers also must be proficient in criteria issued by InterQual and Millman & Robertson, two leading developers of level-of-care guidelines. (Mehallow, 2005)

Telemedicine Healthcare workers

These are healthcare workers who interact with patients via phone or Internet. They advise managed-care subscribers based on physician-developed protocols. Academic medical centers often employ healthcare workers as research assistants to perform telephone consultations with patients participating in clinical trials. Additional academic preparation is usually not required, and many are RNs. (Mehallow, 2005) Some telemedicine is becoming even more expansive and provided by robots, controlled by clinicians at an off site location. Firms such as InTouchHealth based in Santa Barbara assist clinicians to manage care in remote or war-torn locales.

Cruise Ship Healthcare workers

Cruise ships now have floating medical centers on board. These on board care centers resemble urgent care centers and have state of the art equipment, much like an Emergency Department. Healthcare workers see patients both in the center and in cabins if patients are too sick to make it to the medical center. They administer medications, monitor chronic illnesses, and treat emergencies. This role is great for healthcare workers who like to travel and enjoy ER,

ICU and urgent care healthcare. ER experience is usually required, but additional academic preparation is not needed.

Pharmaceutical, Medical Equipment and Supply Educators:

These healthcare workers educate the hospital staff members and physicians who will be using new medical equipment, supplies and pharmaceuticals. Clinical experience in hospitals is usually required, but no additional academic preparation is necessary. Usually this kind of role requires extensive travel and long hours.

School Healthcare workers

If you love working with children and want your summers off, consider school healthcare workers. School healthcare workers do screenings, educate in classrooms, treat sick children and handle emergencies. School healthcare workers also interface with teachers, administrators and parents. Additional training is required. Most school healthcare workers routinely multi-task and are responsible for several schools at a time. This is a great role if you are self-directed and independent.

Occupational Healthcare workers

Occupational and environmental health workers are the specialty practice that provides for and delivers health and safety programs and services to workers, worker populations and community groups. The practice focuses on promotion and restoration of health, prevention of illness and injury and protection from work related and environmental hazards.

In the past two centuries, their responsibilities have expanded immensely to encompass a wide range of job duties, including; case management, Counseling and crisis intervention, Health promotion, legal and regulatory compliance, worker and workplace hazard detection.

Typically, healthcare workers entering the field have a baccalaureate degree in their healthcare specialty and experience in community health, ambulatory care, critical care or emergency healthcare. Certification in occupational and environmental health healthcare workers is highly recommended.

Broadcast Journalists

Healthcare workers can also opt for a broadcasting career. Television anchor and healthcare reporter roles are often filled by healthcare workers. Most healthcare workers in these roles have many years in healthcare and are specialists in at least one area of healthcare. A master's degree is helpful, but not mandatory. This role is a great way to bring your passion for healthcare to the public.

Architectural Building Design/Construction Management

Healthcare workers who enjoy working with the building construction process may have a career niche. Participating in the design of new medical facilities allows healthcare workers to use their clinical mentality, as well as learn skills from the field of architecture and construction management. Assisting architects and construction project managers, healthcare workers can help identify patient flow, systems design, operations logistics and other needs for buildings in development. These types of positions usually require several years of clinical healthcare experience. Healthcare workers can be used as consultants or hired by architectural firms. Healthcare workers can also attend architect programs and become certified as architects, specializing in healthcare facilities.

Healthcare workers Educators and Faculty

Healthcare workers with master's or doctorate degrees are in great demand as faculty at healthcare education programs and schools. The current healthcare faculty shortage is a major contributor to the mushrooming shortage of all types of healthcare workers. Healthcare schools, particularly nursing and pharmacist programs turned away qualified applicants due to a shortage of faculty and resources. Being a healthcare educator allows you to shape the healthcare profession and share your specialty skills and expertise with others.

Healthcare workers with lots of clinical experience have very important skills and perspectives that students and new graduates need to acquire. More faculty members will be required in the future. The shortage of healthcare educators is expected to worsen in coming years as many faculty members retire, particularly in nursing, radiology, and pharmacy programs.

Because clinical experience is a key element of education means healthcare workers who teach don't have to give up patient contact. Teaching in a healthcare workers baccalaureate program does mean earning an advanced degree. Many healthcare workers can find ways to earn an advanced degree without entirely giving up their clinical practice income. Scholarships, forgivable loans and tuition reimbursement programs are all ways to finance becoming a healthcare educator. Financial aid for healthcare workers attending graduate school is available from many sources, including the federal and state governments, hospitals and other healthcare employers, healthcare associations and healthcare schools.

There are online programs to become healthcare educators in some specialties. This enables healthcare workers to fit graduate study into their lives while continuing to work. Perhaps the most difficult obstacle for healthcare workers aspiring to be professors is the salary cut they're likely to experience at the start of their academic careers. The average salary of an emergency room nurse practitioner with a master's degree was nearly $81,000 versus about $60,000 for a healthcare professor with the same academic training, according to a 2003 survey by *Advance for Nurse Practitioners* magazine (Rossman, 2005).However, as they move up the academic ladder in professorial ranks, faculty members with doctoral degrees earn well into six figures.

ADVANCED PRACTICE ROLES

Advanced Practice Healthcare Roles

If you are an experienced healthcare professional, there are a number of opportunities in advanced practice you can pursue. Many of these roles are in nursing, but radiology, dental, and other specialties also have them. There are four categories of advanced practice nursing: healthcare worker practitioners (NPs), certified registered healthcare worker anesthetists (CRNAs), certified healthcare worker-midwives (CNMs) and clinical healthcare worker specialists (CNSes). All require advanced education (typically a master's degree) and clinical experience. After that, certification and state licensing requirements vary.

There are roles in surgical care and making protheses. Dental workers may specialize in making prostheses for teeth such as implants, bridges, and crowns. Radiology technologists can move into nuclear medicine, CT scanning, MRI and other specialties. Additional education varies by state and specialty.

Nurse Practitioners

Nurse Practitioners (NP's) must hold a master's degree and a state license. They are in short supply in many parts of the country and may be an area's only source of primary care, especially in rural settings. NP's are often providing primary healthcare. Their responsibilities include:

- Conducting physicals
- Making diagnoses and providing treatment
- Writing prescriptions
- Managing patients' chronic conditions, such as diabetes and hypertension

NPs must be knowledgeable about prescription medications, be self-directed and self-reliant. They must also know when to call in a physician for consultation or to take over the care of a seriously ill patient. NPs can own their practices; work in hospitals, managed-care organizations and in clinics. To work with physicians in a private practice setting establishing a practice of your own, consider specializing in areas such as women's health or gerontology.

Certified Registered Nurse Anesthetists

Certified Registered Nurse Anesthetists (CRNA's) are among the most highly educated and highly compensated of advanced healthcare worker professionals. In addition, some states are allowing CRNAs to practice without physician supervision. CRNAs work in all settings, from hospitals to private offices. Most states require CRNAs to hold an MSN from an accredited program in the field. CRNAs must also be licensed and certified in their state of practice.

Certified Nurse Midwives

Certified Nurse Midwives (CNMs) provide prenatal and gynecological care to women, deliver babies and provide postpartum care. Most midwife-attended births still occur in hospitals, but CNMs also practice in birthing centers and oversee home births. Many work as solo practitioners or in partnership with an OB/GYN or other CNMs. Most states require CNMs to be RNs, as well as master's prepared.

Clinical Nurse Specialists

Clinical Nurse Specialists (CNSes) are experts in a specialized area of clinical healthcare workers. CNSes can specialize in a specific disease (such as cancer), population (such as women or children), setting (such as an ER), type of care (such as rehab) or type of problem (such as pain). (Rossheim, 2005) CNSes require a master's or PhD and certification to practice as CNSes, and many are also nurse practitioners.

Chief Healthcare Executives

Another option for healthcare workers is to move into the executive suite. With experience in patient care, no one knows better about how all the ancillary services and support patient care needs. Healthcare workers in the Chief Executive role usually serve as healthcare managers and directors prior to taking this type of role. A master's degree in fields such as nursing, health care administration or business administration is required. Some chief healthcare executives move on to become system chief executive or chief operating officers, overseeing the entire healthcare system. Who better to run the place than an experienced healthcare worker?

Dental Lab Technician

Dental technicians make dental prostheses — replacements for natural teeth to help people who have lost some or all of their teeth to eat, chew, talk and smile in a manner that is similar to or better than the way they did before. Technicians work with a variety of materials, as well as sophisticated instruments and equipment, to create dental prostheses — replacements for damaged or missing tooth structure, using small tools and artistic abilities.

Physicians Assistant

Physician assistants (PAs) practice medicine under the direction of physicians and surgeons. They are formally trained to examine patients, diagnose injuries and illnesses, and provide treatment. PAs work in physicians' offices, hospitals, and other healthcare settings. Most work full time. Many physician assistants have a bachelor's degree in a healthcare related field. Then, they must complete an accredited educational program for physician assistants. That usually takes at least 2 years of full-time study and typically leads to a master's degree. All states require physician assistants be licensed and most require a master's degree.

Surgical Assistant/First Assistant

A surgeon's assistant (more commonly referred to as a surgical first assistant or surgical assistant) is a medical or allied health practitioner that provides aide in exposure, hemostasis, and visualization of anatomic structures during the course of a surgical operation. Professionals filling this role come from diverse backgrounds and include medical doctors, surgical residents, surgical physician assistants (PAs), advanced practice registered nurses (such as nurse practitioners), specialized registered nurses (such as registered nurse first assistants or RNFAs), and non-physician surgical first assistant practitioners (SFAs).

Orthotics/Prosthetics

Orthotics and Prosthetics (O&P) is the evaluation, fabrication and custom fitting of artificial limbs and orthopedic braces. O&P is an allied health profession with a variety of exciting employment opportunities available including O&P practitioners, pedorthists, assistants, fitters, and technicians.(2012)

An orthotist is an allied health professional who is specifically trained and educated to provide custom-designed orthoses (external orthopedic braces) and related patient care. A prosthetist is an allied health professional that is specifically trained and educated to provide custom-designed external prostheses (artificial limbs) and related patient care.

An orthotist/prosthetist is an allied health professional that is trained to custom make and fit both orthoses and prostheses. Pedorthics is the design, manufacture, modification of pedorthic devices, to prevent or alleviate foot problems caused by disease, congenital defect, overuse or injury. When credentialed as an O&P professional, one is often referred to as an O&P practitioner. Some of these roles require a master's degree.

Additional roles and job information can be found within 2010-11 edition of the *Occupational Outlook Handbook* include additional roles such as:

Audiologists
Cardiovascular technologists and technicians
Chiropractors
Clinical laboratory technologists and technicians
Dental assistants

Dental hygienists
Dentists
Diagnostic medical sonographers
Dietitians and nutritionists
Emergency medical technicians and paramedics
Home health aides and personal and home care aides
Licensed practical and licensed vocational nurses
Medical and health services managers
Medical assistants
Medical, dental, and ophthalmic laboratory technicians
Medical records and health information technicians
Medical transcriptionists
Nuclear medicine technologists
Nursing and psychiatric aides
Occupational therapist assistants and aides
Occupational therapists
Opticians, dispensing
Optometrists
Pharmacists
Pharmacy technicians and aides
Physical therapist assistants and aides
Physical therapists
Physician assistants
Physicians and surgeons
Podiatrists
Psychologists
Radiation therapists
Receptionists and information clerks
Recreational therapists
Registered nurses
Respiratory therapists
Respiratory therapy technicians
Social and human service assistants

Speech-language pathologists

Surgical technologists

Discussion Questions:

1. Identify non-clinical roles available in hospitals, and the additional education for each role. What is most practical for your specialty? Why?

2. List 3 non-clinical roles outside hospitals.

3. Explain concept of advanced practice nursing and give examples of roles.

4. Identify 3 advanced practice roles for other healthcare specialties and explain each.

5. Choose 4 additional healthcare roles listed in the Job Outlook Handbook and explain:

    a. Role

    b. Work location

    c. Education/experience required

    d. Potential for job opportunities

LIFE AS A NEW
HEALTHCARE GRADUATE

LIFE AS A NEW HEALTHCARE GRADUATE

Chapter Objectives:

1. Identify the process for certification or licensure in your new role.
2. Explain the concept of a novice in healthcare.
3. List 5 things to consider when making your first job selection.
4. Explain the concept of life/work balance, and its importance.

Key terms

Licensure	Preceptor
Certification	New graduate program
Interim permit	Life balance
Job offer	Courtesy
Interview	
Orientation	

Your License

When you successfully complete and graduate from an accredited healthcare program, you must apply for a certificate, interim permit or license. Most professional healthcare roles require either certification or licensure. The process for each healthcare specialty varies by state and healthcare specialty. There is usually a lag time for professional certification or licensure in all healthcare professions. The interim permit is only for RNs and allows you to work as an interim permittee (IP) or interim licensed (IL) RN. Interim permittee status is only in effect from the time you graduate from healthcare school until the time you receive the results of your NCLEX or state board exams. It usually lasts for about three to four months.

Interim permits are issued by your state board of nursing or other specialty. They usually can be obtained online via board web sites or by mail. Interim permits allow nursing school graduates to work as IPs while waiting to take their nursing exams. This means IPs can administer medication, perform procedures and take physician orders under the direct supervision of a licensed registered nurse. This status lasts only until your state board results are made available. You are then either a registered nurse or no longer an IP. If you need to retake the nursing exams (many nurses do), you can apply for an IP again prior to the next exams. Some states have time limits on when you can sit for an exam after being unsuccessful. Most states allow you to take the exams the next time they are offered.

When you obtain your license or certificate, you are a graduate healthcare worker in your specialty. You are entering the healthcare profession as a novice, or someone who has education, but little or no experience. This is your opportunity to learn from more experienced healthcare workers, and not just in your specialty. Hopefully, you will work with staff that is passionate about their profession, as well as kind and willing to help you be successful.

Your First Healthcare Job after Graduation

Many new grads in healthcare professions know before they take their state licensing exams or certification tests where they will be working once they finish school. Most hospitals offer new graduates in many healthcare professions jobs as soon as students have finished school. In most states, nurses are able to work with an interim license until they take and pass their state licensing exam. Other healthcare professions vary by state, specialty and role. You must market yourself to find that first healthcare job. Marketing yourself as a new grad includes standing out from other new grads in your specialty, using your professional network to find out where the jobs are, looking the part of a healthcare professional, and creating a useful resume that will guarantee you an interview.

It is tempting to take the first offer you get as a new grad, but it pays to spend time looking at different facilities prior to accepting any offers. Don't make a quick decision and accept a position after a first interview. You owe it to yourself and your future to conduct your own research about the facilities you interview with. It is always a good idea to interview in more than one healthcare facility. Even if you are certain you only want to work in one specific location or unit, be sure to do multiple interviews in several facilities, so you can make comparisons.

When you conduct your research, be sure to look at internet sites for the facility, look up newspaper and journal articles and review annual reports. Talk to anyone you know who works at a facility you wish to work in. You will learn as much about the facility from those who work there as you will from the individuals that interview you. Your first job sets the stage for the rest of your healthcare career. Choose wisely so you will be able to get grounded in your profession right away. Making a lousy first job choice may mean you need to leave a facility and start over elsewhere.

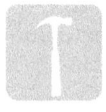 **For your toolkit.... Your first job sets the stage for the rest of your healthcare career. Choose wisely so you will be able to get grounded in your profession right away.**

No matter where you choose to work, be sure you determine what type of orientation and specialty education programs are available for new graduate healthcare workers. Ask specific questions about how long you will orient, if you will be assigned a preceptor, and when you will be "turned loose" to provide patient care in your specialty on your own.

If you are not in an orientation program that is at least a month long (including general orientation days), you will not be adequately prepared to function as a healthcare professional. This will lead to increased stress, feelings of inadequacy, decreased self esteem and self-confidence. It will also affect your clinical competency. Even though you successfully passed healthcare specialty courses, graduated with honors and passed the state licensing/certification exam, you are most likely not ready to practice your specialty by yourself without support from experienced staff.

Some facilities are beginning to offer RN Residencies for new grads. Medical schools have offered MD Residencies for decades. RN Residencies are relatively new, formal education programs that last from three to six months. Residencies offer formal curricula, designated preceptors and mentors, as well as structured clinical experiences on the unit where you will work. Trying to function as a new graduate without the benefit of the skills offered in an RN Residency is much like trying to swim in a pool without having any instruction in swimming skills. I believe that RN Residencies should be and will become the new standard for orientation and training of new graduate nurses. Some other specialties have them as well, including, dental, osteopathy and chiropractic programs.

 **For your toolkit…. RN Residencies should be and will become the new standard for orientation and training of new graduate nurses.**

Wherever you work, you will need a comprehensive immersion program that is designed to transition newly graduated healthcare workers from a student to a safe, competent professional. The many facets of a program allow facilities to prepare competent, safe and confident healthcare workers, and simultaneously manage complex operational issues such as recruitment, retention, and self confidence. A program research and evaluation process allows facilities to statistically quantify operational risk of new grad turnover and lack of organizational loyalty. (Versant, 2005)

You should determine if there is an evaluation that provides the organization with analytical results that allow proactive monitoring of loyalty and potential turnover risks (Versant, 2005). If you have an opportunity to work in a facility that has an RN Residency (especially the Versant model), sign up! It will be a great new grad transition experience, and you will likely stay in that environment for at least several years.

If a healthcare worker residency or orientation program is not available at the facility you wish to work at, ask about formal orientation and precepting options. You definitely want to work at a facility with a formal orientation program. You will have to attend facility orientation with all new employees.

Healthcare workers doing direct patient care usually will receive additional orientation and clinical nurses even more. However, once those are completed, you will still need orientation to the role of your professional healthcare specialty. Ask the interviewer how that is accomplished in this particular facility. If they cannot explain an organized and formalized process or program to you, and do not assign you a preceptor/resource person for a minimum of three months, reconsider working there.

Many new grads get frustrated and leave their healthcare specialty role within the first year of graduation. This happens because their orientation was poor or non-existent. It is not reasonable to expect someone right out of school be competent, safe and confident with 2 weeks of hospital orientation and nothing else. Don't sell yourself, your specialty or your patients short. Insist on formal orientation and an individual preceptor before you accept a new grad position in any healthcare specialty.

Having a Life and a Career: Achieving Life Balance

Because your first job sets the tone for your first professional healthcare experience, it is critical that you are well prepared for it. In addition to a formal orientation program as discussed previously, you must also find a way to balance your life. Healthcare is a stressful profession, so you need some self care strategies to make the most of your life and your healthcare role.

Most importantly, when you start a new job, remember you do not have to know everything. It is a myth that healthcare employers expect new graduate staff to know all there is to know about being a professional whatever. Even experienced staff starts out as a novice when they go into a new role. It is *okay* to not know things. You are not expected to know everything. Remind yourself of that every day!

Employers do expect healthcare workers to deliver safe and competent care to patients. That is why choosing a job with a formal orientation program or a RN Residency is so important. There is a steep learning curve for all newly hired or licensed/certified healthcare workers. How fast you learn is individualized and different for each person. You are not expected to know everything. Asking for help will not label you as incompetent or a burden. Ask for help *before* you are drowning. You are not expected to be perfect, but rather to know what you don't know. It is also important for you to ask questions about situations and care practices you are not familiar with. You are responsible for telling your supervisor if you are not trained or have never performed a specific skill that you are asked to do as a new healthcare worker.

Healthcare is profession where safety and precision are significant. Policies and procedures exist to ensure that nothing is taken for granted and care is provided in the safest way possible. Policies and procedures may seem cumbersome and time consuming, but they are created as safeguards to protect patients. It is crucial that you ask for and follow facility procedures and policies to avoid errors that may endanger patients, families or fellow staff members. The reality check that occurs after you make a mistake that significantly affects a patient outcome is not the way to start your healthcare career.

Because you can't know everything, it is important to know where to find the information you need. Cultivate resources and use them. Internet web sites, policy and procedure manuals, textbooks, "How to be a new grad" booklets and pocket guides are all useful tools to gather information. Preceptors are often designated for new grads or experienced healthcare workers in a new position. You should request one if you are not assigned one as a new grad. You can consult other staff besides your preceptor to mentor or coach you. Find an experienced healthcare professional in your specialty that you trust and use him/her as a guide when you are unsure of how to proceed.

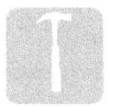 **For your toolkit....Find a staff member you can trust to be your mentor or coach. Use this person as a guide when you are unsure of how to proceed.**

It is also a good idea to find someone to answer questions when you move to a new unit or shift. When you switch to the night shift, which many new grads do during their first year, you need advice. It is really helpful to have someone who already works nights tell you how they survive the hours, manage their family, sleeping strategies and other tips. If you move or float to another unit, find a person that seems approachable and ask how they suggest you begin. Unfortunately, not everyone will be friendly and helpful, but you will find most staff eager to share their experiences and ideas.

Common courtesy and graciousness will go a long way when you are new on a job. They are as important as your clinical specialty skills to your success. "Please" and "thank you" are not out of style and will make experienced staff more willing to assist you with questions. As Joan Duncan Oliver says, "Kindness is one of the most undervalued commodities…" (Hill, 1998) Be pleasant to everyone, and try to avoid "choosing" a clique in your new workplace. It is likely that there will be work groups or cliques already formed in your new unit. Be careful about being drawn into one, especially the special interest groups that are negative or non-productive.

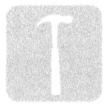 **For your toolkit…. Common courtesy and graciousness are as important as your clinical skills for success**

Try and meet new people every day. Don't be shy in the cafeteria and introduce yourself to staff from other departments. Find out what their role is in your facility. Some facilities even have "welcome programs". These programs ask that other staff introduce themselves to new staff and explain where they work. This strategy is a great way to meet new people and discover resources in other departments.

Keep in mind while it is a great idea to reach out to work with others, you need to maintain healthy boundaries for yourself. As the "newbie" you will be asked by other staff to work a weekend, take an extra shift or to perform other tasks. Don't let other staff take advantage of you. If you wish to work extra that's great. But if you would rather not, then don't get sucked into their situation. Remember it is okay to maintain your boundaries and individuality and to say no.

You will be learning many new things each day in your first job as a healthcare professional. Consider journaling your ideas, problems, solutions and strategies each day as a way of reflecting as well as storing information.

If you used reflective journaling in your healthcare program, you are already familiar with the format for doing journaling. You don't need anything fancy to write in or special writing talents. Just write about your shift, thoughts, feelings and ideas. It is a great stress reducer.

Remember, you have been trained to be a problem solver and to use critical thinking skills. While healthcare demands precision and specificity, there are also many areas that are unclear, with differences of opinions as well as gray areas. You will find that even the experts disagree on specific procedures and processes to complete healthcare tasks. You will likely develop your own opinions and ideas once you have some patient care experience. Focus on critical thinking strategies and problem solving skills to stay balanced.

Last but definitely not least, you need to take care of yourself. You cannot care for others effectively without caring for yourself first. This is true while you are caring for patients, raising children and interacting with family members, spouses or significant others. You need to identify several ways you can disconnect from your work. Do something– yoga, meditation, walking the dog, listening to music, baths– whatever it takes to let you unplug and reflect.

Also plan some alone time for yourself. Alone time isn't selfish or being irresponsible. Keep in mind that alone time is doing something for your soul space. Alone time is not going to the grocery store, doing laundry or commuting to work. Make an appointment with yourself and do something renewing. You deserve some time alone without justifying it by multitasking. Dr. Phil (McGraw) says that quality alone time must nourish your relationship with yourself. His rule of thumb is "If you were doing the same activity with your kids, would it nourish your relationship with them?" (2004) Watching a movie may be enjoyable, but it doesn't bring you closer to the person you are sitting next to. Since alone time is about building a relationship with yourself, the same is true. Everyone is different. You don't have to sit alone and stare at the walls. Find a way to look inward. Write in a journal. Create a life plan. Create a career plan. Take a walk. Have a massage. Do whatever works for you to focus inwardly and renew yourself.

Healthcare is a rewarding profession, but it is stressful and takes energy out of your body and soul. Be sure you refill your "pot of energy" and your soul space to keep yourself healthy and able to provide care. Finding private time for yourself will refill your soul and renew your spirit. Remember, that being a healthcare professional is more than being competent. It is about being of service. In order to be of service, you must have energy to work with.

Discussion Questions:

1. Explain why a formal orientation program is so important to your first year of success.

2. Identify ways to balance your life and work.

3. Discuss why mentors and/or coaches are so important.

4. Describe in detail the licensure/certification process for your particular specialty.

Case Studies:

1. Candy is a new radiology technologist. She has applied at the facility in her community. They promise her an orientation, a "buddy" and a reasonable salary. What questions should she ask about this offer? Why? What is missing from the offer?

2. Mary is a new grad RN. She started on a medical-surgical floor following graduation. She attended hospital general orientation, and an additional week of clinical orientation. She has a resource RN. Mary is frightened, exhausted, and wants to quit. What would you tell her? Why?

PROFESSIONAL ADVOCACY

"A healthy population is one of our nation's most important assets. To protect this asset, health care must be at the forefront of our society's consciousness. Without coherent state and national health care policies, the heath of our communities and the existence of our hospitals are in jeopardy." (ACNL, 1995)

PROFESSIONAL ADVOCACY

Chapter Objectives:

1. Define professional advocacy and explain why it is important.
2. List 4 ways to be a professional advocate.
3. List 8 characteristics of remarkable employees.
4. Compare and contrast embellishment vs. integrity.
5. Explain who is responsible for healthcare worker retention and why.
6. List 4 retention strategies for healthcare workers in your specialty and why they might be effective.
7. Identify key survival strategies during turbulent times.
8. List 3 risks and 3 rewards for using survival strategies

Key terms

Political advocacy   professional advocacy
Remarkable employee   Integrity
Retention   Nurturing young workers
Survival strategies   Professional networking

Nurturing Our Young

There are important functions in being a healthcare advocate. It is part of our professional responsibility and part of being of service to do these tasks throughout our career. Some examples are listed below:

- **Nurture those who come after you.** Some health professions such as nurses are famous for "eating their young." That is such a disturbing phrase, but so true. Let's change it to "nurturing our young." It is our responsibility to coach and mentor healthcare staff less experienced than us. Be kind to healthcare students and new grads. You never know when *they* might end up taking care of *you!*

- **Feed the machine.** Talk about your career in healthcare and encourage others to join the professions in the industry. Participate in the career days at your local schools and volunteer to talk about your specialty role in your community.

- **Be a healthcare worker 24/7.** Identify and introduce yourself as a healthcare worker whenever you meet a new person. Role model professional conduct, clothing and behavior whenever you are in public. It is tough to be depicted as a bimbo if you never act like one.

- **Let go of old issues.** We don't have to agree on everything to work together as a profession or industry. The proper credentials for entry into nursing practice, how much training a phlebotomist should have or other professions are not silver bullet issues. We need to advocate for all the healthcare professions, and each other.

- **Cultivate your experiences and skills.** Seek out opportunities to learn and new things. Every skill you acquire gets added to your personal career toolkit that you take with you from job to job. It can never be too full!

- **Become a lifelong learner.** Continue to take classes and advance your professional knowledge. Commit to expanding your learning and long term career development.

- **Use staff to their maximum potential.** It doesn't matter whether you are a manager or not. Chances are you work with someone that you delegate tasks to. Encourage them to expand their knowledge. Ensure you expect the best they can be and give them tasks that allow that behavior to emerge.

- **Nurture yourself emotionally and spiritually.** Because healthcare is about being of service, remember to take care of yourself. Balance your life–feed your soul and your heart so you can continue giving to others.

 **For your toolkit....Experienced healthcare workers must nurture their young!**

Be a Remarkable Employee

In one of the most important roles in healthcare, you have a chance to be outstanding. As a healthcare professional, you are likely reliable, dependable, proactive, tenacious, with strong leadership and excellent communication skills. However, there are some leaders that hit the next level. If you have worked for one, you know what I mean. Even thought these qualities may not appear on performance appraisals, they make a major impact on success and the organization.

Jeff Haden notes there are eight qualities of remarkable employees: (www.inc.com/jeff-haden). These qualities include:

1. They ignore job descriptions and think on their feet in spite of shifting priorities. They do whatever it takes to get the job done.

2. They are eccentric with unusual personalities and quirky behaviors that are not afraid to be different. This allows them to stretch boundaries and challenge the status quo.

3. They know when to be a part of the team. When a major challenge or stressful situation occurs they fit seamlessly into the team.

4. They publicly praise. Praise from a boss feels good, and even better from a peer.

5. They privately complain. They bring up sensitive issues privately to avoid a firestorm in a group setting.

6. They speak when others won't. They have an innate feel for issues and often ask questions when others won't. Have you ever asked a tough question in a group and watched others around you nodding their heads in agreement?

7. They have self-motivation and a burning drive for effectiveness and success of the team.

8. They always tinker with the processes and systems to make them better.

You may be blessed to have several of these folks in your organization. You may even work for one. It gives us all something to strive for. Are you willing to be remarkable?

Embellishment vs. Integrity

Many of us saw the recent news of the Yahoo CEO Scott Thompson who resigned in May, 2012 over a "little white lie" on his resume from years ago. Although it was called an "inadvertent error," this was a huge professional blunder by Thompson; one that cost him his job, and his company more bad publicity and tumbling stock values.

It is tempting for everyone to embellish a bit on their resume, especially as you move up the healthcare leadership ladder. We all want to look good to potential interviewers, our peers and our subordinates. However, we also answer to a higher source: our patients. Several healthcare professions are among the most trusted professions. (http://nursinglink.monster.com/education/articles/3269-registered-nurses-most-trusted-profession). Can you really afford to lose that trust?

One of the definitions of professionalism listed in Wikipedia is" a high standard of professional ethics, behavior and work activities while carrying out one's profession..."(http://en.wikipedia.org/wiki/Professionalism). As professionals, we are held to a high standard of integrity, honor, role modeling and integrity. Take a look at your resume or CV now and be sure it is accurate and honest down to the last detail. It matters to all of us who have been graciously granted public trust by the healthcare education we earned.

Professional Retention

Retention for those professions experiencing long standing shortages is the responsibility of *every* healthcare professional. The most well known shortages are of pharmacists and registered nurses. There are plenty of innovative strategies being suggested by nursing executives, school directors and faculty. There are different answers for different regions of the country, but we all need to focus on the same goal. Start looking at ways to increase healthcare faculty positions and hire qualified individuals in your local community. Joint appointments of managers and clinical staff to faculty positions are one way to partner between hospitals and schools for healthcare education. Evaluation of part time and shared faculty positions for a variety of healthcare education opportunities will increase enrollment of students and eliminate waiting lists. Healthcare faculty will need assistance with creating other clinical faculty opportunities with local hospital clinical staff. Local healthcare administrators can be used as paid guest lecturers. Ask your local hospitals to sponsor skills labs through regional hospital organizations.

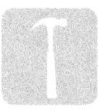 **For your toolkit... Healthcare retention is the responsibility of every healthcare professional.**

Mandated staffing ratios and deepening shortages in some healthcare professions require solutions and strategies different than those used in the past. While there is no one magic recipe to fix the limited number of student slots in these healthcare programs, there is one simple answer for the college administrators and chancellors. Get started. Step up to the plate and do something! Healthcare staff in both service and academia stand ready to assist, but cannot do this without college and university chancellor impetus and input to expand educational capacity.

Healthcare facilities need to commit to several strategies to assist with reversing these shortages in their geographic regions. Effective strategies include the implementation of magnet characteristics as outlined in The Magnet Recognition Program®. This program was developed by the American Nurses Credentialing Center to recognize health care organizations that provide the very best in nursing care and uphold the tradition within nursing of professional nursing practice. There are also workplace components that improve hiring potential listed on several recruitment websites.

Additional retention strategies include utilizing foreign-trained healthcare staff in US hospitals. There is a decreasing trend to recruit foreign nurses and healthcare workers as replacement staff as too expensive. However, there is foreign-trained staff currently residing in the U.S. To accommodate foreign healthcare staff who currently reside in the U.S., collaboration with local community colleges can encourage their maintenance of wait lists these specific classes for all healthcare specialties. When there's an opening due to student attrition, a foreign trained healthcare professional can be allowed to fill it.

Offering healthcare residencies to new graduates upon hiring has been demonstrated as the best retention strategy by far (2004). Other focuses include expansion of compressed salary grids, offering retention bonuses instead of sign on/recruitment bonuses. Hospitals can host job shadowing and tour days at facilities for high school and college students considering a healthcare career. It has been demonstrated by several research studies that facilities that provide formal education, valuing and compensating staff preceptors and mentors within organizations have more satisfied employees and higher retention rates.

Retention strategies also must be specifically cultivated for "Boomer staff". As they enter their fifties, many Baby Boom-era healthcare professionals can no longer cope with active clinical care. Creating and offering other employment opportunities within hospitals for staff no longer able to manage the physical demands of bedside clinical care would go a long way to keeping "Boomers" working instead of retiring. Using "Boomers" for coaches, mentors, preceptors and educators would let them provide valuable experience to new healthcare staff that need compassionate and kind oversight. Facilities can implement shorter shift options, including 4-6 hr shifts, as many older staff members cannot handle 12 hours shifts physically. Job sharing or flexible or self-scheduling options are also staff-retaining options.

Hospitals can also provide pre-retirement information sessions to discuss reassignment options. These non-clinical options could include case management, patient advocacy, education, quality improvement or mentoring. Keeping older healthcare staff in patient care setting as mentors is a valuable resource to less experienced staff and increases retention of both older and newer healthcare professionals.

Healthcare systems may want to evaluate the feasibility of utilizing a deferred pension fund jointly with employment, as public service agencies have done throughout the country. Police and fire services facing massive retirements from employees hired after the Vietnam War who were ready to retire, developed deferred retirement options and plans (DROP). These plans allowed police and firefighters to retire from their positions if they had twenty or more years of service (2010). They could then reapply for their same job, earning both a salary and pension at the same time. This strategy encouraged many police and firefighters to remain in the workforce instead of retiring. Most plans have a maximum enrollment time of five years, but that still helps with retention of important public service staff.

Facilities could consider hiring aging healthcare staff as Retention Specialists. Their roles/responsibilities could include meeting with aging staff, facilitating problem solving and being empathetic listeners. They would serve as a mediator and mentor resources. In addition, this role could try to get retired healthcare staff back into facilities that have left by attempting to resolve personal concerns and creating innovative solutions for older personnel. This type of role could have a significant impact and can save healthcare staff while limiting vacancies. It's win-win for the healthcare facilities that embrace these types of retention ideas. The aging healthcare workers remain employed and the hospital improves staffing with experienced professionals.

Healthcare facilities also need to remember how important having effective and competent managers is to retention. 50% of employee satisfaction comes from their relationship with their boss (Kaye & Jordan-Evans). Research shows that the quality of the relationship between a boss and subordinate is a primary predictor of intentions to remain in a job or facility (Thomas).

An investment in strengthening an organization's leaders- from senior executives to middle managers to team leaders-pays off in all sorts of ways, but particularly in attracting and retaining employees.(Buckingham et al) Those hospitals that had measures in place to hold managers accountable for retention tended to experience lower turnover rates. Accountability measures can include incorporating retention efforts into the managers' performance appraisal process, bonuses for taking action related to turn-over or achieving a qualitative or quantitative change in the turnover rate, and periodic review of employee satisfaction in the manager's specific service area. (Abrams, 2002)

The bottom line is that retention must be the new emphasis in healthcare facilities. Recruitment strategies must continue, but not to the exclusion of retaining competent healthcare staff who want to keep working. Healthcare workers must be seen as what they truly are– a precious resource that is the mainstay of hospital care.

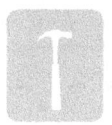 **For your toolkit... Retention must be the new emphasis in healthcare facilities.**

Survival Strategies during turbulent times

All healthcare professionals need survival strategies during turbulent times. Every staff member deals with difficulties in a healthcare organization. With the evolving shortages and other challenges of healthcare, there are more and more opportunities to feel like you are barely surviving. Here are some strategies for survival during those tough times.

Survival Skills:

- Understand rightsizing of management and workers
- Eliminate duplication of tasks and people
- Cross train whenever possible
- Eliminate fragmentation and departmental barriers
- Minimize non productive time
- Determine ways to move services to customers and patients
- Find ways to measure and reward customer satisfaction and quality
- Streamline patient processes, systems and documentation
- Be seen as a leader/supporter of organization mission and values
- Epitomize the characteristics of an indispensable nurse

There are both risks and rewards for using these survival strategies.

Risks	Rewards
Inability to be positive all the time	Employment
Increased stress	Empowerment seized
Lack of security	Increased self confidence
Ambiguity	Increased value to your organization
May be seen as traitor by colleagues	Personal growth
Feel "caught in the middle"/isolated	Opportunities for innovation
Crisis oriented mentality	Expanding horizons and job choices
Changing relationships	Pride
Failure	Professionalism

Traditional behaviors and socialization of healthcare staff also exist. These perceptions are often reality. I list them here to identify that reality without judgment:

Females:
- Be dependent
- Take care of others
- "Be there" 24/7
- Be nice
- Don't be selfish
- Be collaborative at your expense
- Be warm, loving, nurturing
- Don't bother anyone
- Don't say no
- Don't get angry
- Be thin, gorgeous and have great clothes
- Keep family traditions
- Learn to "read" others and anticipate their needs (codependence!)
- Always cooperate, no mater what
- Don't act smarter than boys
- It is ok to cry if you are upset

Males

- Be independent
- Be aggressive
- Express anger, but no other emotions
- Never cry
- Keep your feelings to yourself
- View power and control as career success
- Know that female role is to nurture males
- Regard home as just a place to relax with no accountability
- Be direct and straightforward
- Be goal oriented and future oriented
- Be smarter than women and let them know it
- Give directions
- Be well built, muscular and not fat

Healthcare means being of service to others

"The real essences of nursing, as of any fine art, lies not in the mechanical details of execution, nor yet in the dexterity of the performer, but in the creative imagination, the sensitive spirit, and the intelligent understanding lying back of these techniques and skills. Without these, nursing may become a highly skilled trade, but it cannot be a profession or a fine art. All the rituals and ceremonials which our modern worship of efficiency may devise, and all our elaborate scientific equipment will not save us if the intellectual and spiritual elements in our art are subordinated to the mechanical, and if the means come to be regarded as more important than ends." Stewart, 1929

Although the saying above applies to nursing, it relates to all healthcare roles. Healthcare is a service field. While the care and tasks we perform for patients are highly technical and sophisticated, all healthcare roles are about being of service. Patients are the customers (as well as physicians) and there is a responsibility of serving the customers to the best of our ability. Do not mistake this concept for taking verbal or physical abuse from physicians. That is not the same thing.

Customer service is about being of service. Healthcare staff uses characteristics like persuasion, influence, courteous, honoring patients' feelings/needs, being present for the patient both inside and out, listening, and interpreting non verbal cues, intuition.

Being of service means dealing with angry patients, families, staff and physicians. There are numerous changes that occur in a healthcare setting that affect front line staff. Some staff members can roll with the changes and not take them personally. Others have more difficulty separating their personal feelings from the changes in the organization. These folks tend to get angry and take it out on whoever they work most closely with.

 **For your toolkit…Healthcare is about being of service.**

Being of service is stress producing and exhausting. Be sure you take care of yourself, as outlined in the chapter on balancing your life. It is important to let go of work and patient care issues after hours and find ways to take care of your body, mind and soul. The alternative to not taking care of you is burnout, professional malaise and compassion fatigue. There has been much written about burnout and compassion fatigue. It is preventable. Be as caring and a strong advocate for yourself as you would a patient. Don't deny the need you have to have a balanced life, emotional stability and a centered, peaceful soul. Learn ways to monitor your own health state. Honor your feelings and physical sensations. As my dear friend Katheryn Kray says, "When you have had enough you'll know." That way you can do something to change things. Keep in mind that when you feel bad; it is bad and you need to take care of yourself.

Graciousness is Mandatory

We all know how it feels to be treated rudely at a meeting, have someone not follow-up as expected or promised, or feeling like someone took advantage of us as a professional contact. No matter what happens to you-mergers, acquisitions, downsizing, layoffs, graciousness is mandatory. Rude behavior and unprofessional etiquette have no place in the work setting.

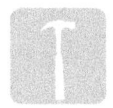

For your toolkit... Graciousness is Mandatory

When you meet someone new, make eye contact and say hello. When you are in a room full of people, be sure your attitude is one of meeting everyone as opposed to "What can you do for me?" Make sure you meet people because of inviting eye contact, not because you are shopping for important people. Make sure you have effective listening skills. Keep in mind that active listening is more than just not talking. There are lots of resources available to enhance your skills if you frequently find yourself asking people to repeat themselves.

If you promise to assist or get back to someone, leave a voicemail or email with the information requested within a few days. To make someone wait longer is sloppy and unprofessional. Develop your own system to keep track of the business cards you get so they are not lost or forgotten. I usually write notes to myself on the back of business cards reminding me of how I met that person, what their children's names are and the name of their secretary. The notes will help you remember important information as well as remember when to follow-up.

Abuse in the Work Place

I am disappointed to report that as an employee, consultant, and monster.com expert, I have heard about many incidents of on the job abuse by physicians, coworkers, supervisors and patients. These incidents run the gamut from verbal abuse to throwing an operating room light fixture. Abuse of any sort is a very serious issue and should not be tolerated. Nurses sometimes become accustomed to abuse, and therefore it is ignored, avoided or excused. Many healthcare staff believe they are powerless to combat abuse, or they perceive that no one in their organization really cares about its impact. You do have some options to take care of yourself and avoid abusive situations.

Almost all organizations now have specific policies against harassment, abusive behavior and hostile work environments. These policies are very strict, so familiarize yourself with what exists in your facility and what the reporting process is. You must also immediately report any case of abuse to your supervisor verbally. You may also need to create a written report of the incident, depending on the circumstances. If your supervisor does not respond or dismisses the incident, report it again through your human resources department.

Keep personal written records of the event and your reporting attempts. Keep an extra copy of that documentation at home, in what I like to call a "hot" file. That way, if anything happens to the work copies, there are others available. Use your hot file to document any potentially difficult or legal incident that occurs in the workplace, including abusive behavior. Be sure to also follow your facility's required official documentation processes. Document, both at work and in your personal hot file, the incident, whether it was isolated or ongoing, what occurred, the date, time, witnesses, who said what to who, and what actions you took.

If the abuser is a manager who oversees others, that makes things a bit more complicated, but no more tolerable. When a manager is abusive, other supervisors and coworkers may choose to ignore or tolerate the situation. When bad behavior is overlooked, that behavior is supported and encouraged at some level—even if we don't mean to do so. In the event of an encounter with an abusive manager or supervisor, immediately call others to the scene to witness the behavior. There is strength in numbers, and you may be able to persuade your colleagues to join forces to stop the abuse.

It is all too common to hear of a physician screaming at a nurse who asked about not being able to read illegible orders or not accepting a patient because the unit is full or being contacted when a patient is unstable. In my experience, abusive physicians are far more common than abusive healthcare staff. My worst experience was having a physician scream at me about being incompetent as a director in front of the patient, the family and several employees. Because he was so loud, every one on the unit heard his ranting. I decided that day that I would not let his behavior go unreported. I told the physician that it was clear to me he was very angry. I said I was unwilling to be spoken to like that, and when he calmed down I would be happy to meet with him about his concerns. Then, I did the hardest thing of all with my heart in my throat. I turned around and walked back to my office some distance away. Amazingly enough, he stopped yelling, finished up with the patient, and came to talk with me about 30 minutes later. His concerns were actually quite valid. It was his approach that was totally unacceptable. I did report his behavior through the medical staff reporting mechanisms, and he apologized to me and the staff. As far as I know, he never did it again to any other staff member in that facility.

The next time you are approached by a screaming physician or other individual, think about stopping the behavior for your sake, as well as your co-workers. You might attempt to confront the person in private and inform him/her you do not wish to be spoken to in that manner, and advise him/her that you will be forced to report him to the medical direc-tor or department chairman—whatever your policy dictates. You may also ask for an apology, although in my experience, this tends to inflame these sorts even more.

You could also provide the offending physician, your supervisor and the medical director or chairman with a copy of at least one of the several articles written in the past several years about physicians' abusive behavior being a contributing factor to the nursing and other healthcare shortages. I'm sorry to report there are a lot of them listed on the internet.

Encourage your facility to adopt a physician Code of Conduct. When physicians understand that their behavior is contributing to the severe short-age of some types of healthcare workers (particularly nurses) in this country, most are happy to participate in the solution instead of being part of the prob-lem. Create a committee composed of nurses, physicians, other healthcare professionals and administrators to develop a Code of conduct, a physician abuse policy and the mechanisms to curtail this type of behavior in your facility.

For your toolkit...Physician abuse of healthcare staff is a workplace retention issue.

The other group that tends to get abusive towards healthcare staff is patients. I have had two experiences of this in my clinical career and both times were very scary. I had a patient in the ER break a glass IV bottle (yes, it was in those days) and threaten to kill me with the jagged edge of the broken bottle. He was high on PCP, and the police were summoned. I ended up on the floor with him on top of me screaming. Fortunately, I wasn't hurt and the police responded quickly, but it was frightening. The other incident involved a father whose child died in ICU and could not contain his anger at the death of his only son. He threatened all the nurses who cared for his son with a gun. He calmed down quickly and never touched anyone, but the staff was really shook up.

Patients who attempt to assault staff are dangerous and should be dealt with immediately. Employers are responsible, and legally accountable to make responsible efforts to protect workers from workplace hostility. If you are assaulted by a patient, secure yourself and the other patients. Most facilities have a security code page for the operators to use. Once the situation is controlled, report the event to your supervisor verbally, and prepare a written report as well. Submit a report to the patient's physician as well. It may be that any patient who throws things or attempts to physically assault a healthcare worker could have a psychiatric disorder.

Most facilities have rules and policies about abusive behavior, but the reporting of these events is not common. Enforcing the rules usually only occurs when an incident comes up, so many staff members are not aware of the process prior to an event. Many staff have decided to tolerate abuse which only perpetuates the problem. Less tolerance of abusive behavior in the workplace will slowly force the behaviors to change. Protect yourself and your colleagues by taking appropriate action when these events occur. Taking care of yourself reflects your value as a human being and improves the workplace for everyone.

articles on abuse

- http://www.findarticles.com/p/articles/mi_m0FSL/is_3_74/ai_80159514

- http://www.usnews.com/usnews/health/articles/020617/archive_021640.htm

- http://xnet.kp.org/permanentejournal/winter04/pal.html

- http://healthcare.monster.com/nursing/articles/verbalabuse/

- http://www.nursingcenter.com/library/JournalArticle.asp?Article_ID=278949

- http://www2.nurseweek.com/Articles/article.cfm?AID=14548

- http://educate.crisisprevention.com/WorkplaceViolence.html?code=ITG006SCWE&src=Pay-Per-Click&gclid=CIHuwJGTq7ACFccBRQodT09-XQ

- http://www.lni.wa.gov/safety/research/files/bullying.pdf

- http://counselingoutfitters.com/vistas/vistas05/Vistas05.art62.pdf

- http://www.workplacebullying.org/individuals/problem/definition/

- http://suite101.com/article/emotional-abuse-in-the-workplace-a73977

- http://educate.crisisprevention.com/WorkplaceViolence.html?code=ITG006SCWE&src=Pay-Per-Click&gclid=CMLmtvyTq7ACFQF6hwodSUVVVg

The Importance of Networking

Networking with other professionals is a process of creating links to obtain information, influence and power. It is the process of exchanging information between strategically placed individuals who have access to ideas and other people. (Turner, 1996) Networking is what allows people to become connectors.

Connectors are people that link ideas together between groups (Gladwell, 2004). Knowing a connector is valuable to your career and using them well is priceless!

Healthcare professionals don't often recognize the value of using a professional network to enhance your career. Some folks believe that asking for help means that you cannot do it on your own. There is nothing wrong with asking for help to achieve something. Many of us perceive we will be using people. Folks who enjoy coaching and mentoring actually liked being asked for help. If you have received value from mentoring, coaching or using a network, be sure you offer it to others. It is up to those of us with experience to assist the staff coming along behind us so they too can be successful. It is not only a way to be of service, but part of our professional responsibility.

 **For your toolkit... Knowing a connector is valuable to your career and using them well is priceless!**

The process of developing contacts and networking will assist you in accomplishing career goals, problem solving and advancing your career. It has often been said by management gurus that 75% of job offers occur because of networking (NOT answering ads for interviews). This fact demonstrates that networking with other professionals is critical to your career success. Networking can be done in social situations, with family and friends or at business meetings. It requires a conscious commitment of time, energy and resources.

Networking is a long term strategy for professional and career advancement. The rewards do not occur quickly and the benefits often take years to be realized. I once met a hospital administrator during an interview for a job I really didn't want, and spoke to her about my career goals. I shared what I wanted to do, and how I thought I could get there. She kept my business card and called me two years later when she had the kind of job I wanted. I worked with her for several years and still keep in contact.

Creating these linkages and networking with professionals is an active practice. It cannot be accomplished by default. You must dedicate energy and schedule time to do it. I find my most successful networking opportunities occur over meals. It is relaxing to meet someone in a restaurant and talk with them about my goals. The value of the advice I get always outweighs what I paid for our meal. If you invite someone out to eat with you for the purpose of networking, always pick up the tab for the meal.

Networking can help you accomplish professional goals if you identify your own career goals and share them with mentors and coaches. You must create, initiate and cultivate contacts. To use this linkage method, you must identify existing networks of colleagues and appropriate methods to achieve your goals and career advancement. Net working requires effort and thought on your part. If you do not put in the time and energy, you will not have a successful outcome.

Some folks are unclear as to what constitutes networking. These activities are all part of active networking:

- Making phone calls just to chat–even when you don't need anything
- Talking with colleagues about open positions you think they might be interested in, or industry news (not gossip) that could be helpful to their role function
- Promptly returning phone calls from colleagues if they request information from you
- Writing thank you notes to colleagues for information they have shared with you or advice received
- Phoning a colleague to ask for assistance in solving a problem
- Inviting colleagues or contacts out for lunch

Strategies for successful networking include participation in a professional organization and subscribing to at least one professional journal/magazine. This kind of investment in your future will also assist you in deciding if you need further education, specialized training or more subscriptions. It is important to keep up to date and informed in your specialty and about healthcare changes.

We have all been on the receiving end of a "networking nightmare." Examine your own networking etiquette to see if you need to make some changes. It is inappropriate to network with the attitude "how can you help me? "You know the type. They scan name tags to see who will be useful to talk to and skip past those whose job titles seem uninteresting. Meet someone because of your inviting eye contact. It's tacky to shop for important people.

When you first meet someone, don't blab on with self importance. Practice a short introduction that states who you are and what you do. Try not to give just your job title, as if it explains everything. Job titles mean different things in different industries, so be specific.

Create a system for following up with people you meet. Design a filing system to keep track of the business cards you receive. Use your smart phone or write notes on the back that will help you recall important information or remind you to follow up. Use voicemail, email or a personal note to contact someone you promised to respond to. It's tacky to fail to contact someone, so always keep your promise to contact them.

Join at least one professional or business organization, so you can begin building a reputation as a doer or a donor or both. You will be seen as someone who is serious about your career, your contacts and your industry and not just a short timer. Be sure to send a thank you note or make a thank you call when someone has helped you. Doing so sends the message that you are gracious and not just a taker. Being gracious makes people want to help you again.

Don't wait until you have a crisis to start networking. Most folks wait for some drastic change in their professional life to make contact. A layoff or relocation can cause panic enough. Build a web of contacts BEFORE you need them, and when things are going well. Be sure to network with those people who are just starting out. It is tempting to only "network up", but in healthcare you never know where they will be in a few years. That is especially true in healthcare.

Being available to network is crucial. If you are always too busy or never follow through, colleagues will stop making plans with you. To successfully network, you must be visible in the nursing community. To be visible takes time and energy. As you develop networks, mentors and coaches, remember to say thank you for what you learn, information that is shared and never broach a confidence or private information.

Political Advocacy

Many healthcare issues that affect our communities are also social policy issues. Healthcare workers are in a unique position to educate politicians about health issues and affect change. It is important for every healthcare worker to become politically active.

Political influence is necessary to direct state and federal legislation that affect the operation of our health care delivery system. Providing knowledge about health and populations into the political process is an important role for care givers. Because healthcare workers have strong connections to their community and are employed in all parts of the health continuum; they become crucial to influencing state and federal legislators as volunteer political advocates.

For your toolkit...Every healthcare worker should be a political advocate for healthcare issues.

As a healthcare professional, you have both skills and expertise to educate legislators and citizens that are served and employed in your community. Politics and health care delivery systems get more interrelated as pressures for cost-effective, accessible and quality health services become part of the political agenda. Federal, state and local fiscal management problems have necessitated greater government involvement in health care to control spending for public health care programs. The government must also assure that fiscal limitations of health providers do not deny access to care for people who need it.

Other factors also are changing the environment in tandem with changes to public health care programs. The number of uninsured and underinsured persons has steadily climbed, adding more to the already strained hospitals in the form of uncompensated care. An aging population, higher labor costs, new technologies, and labor shortages are additional factors aggravating the current situation.

Get informed about the health policy issues in your state and community. Learn about the legislative process. Reference materials specifically for healthcare workers on health policy advocacy are available from many professional organizations including the American Nurses' Association, American Physical Therapy Association, American Registry of Radiology Technologists, National Pharmacist Organization and others. Participate in public meetings and hearings on important issues. Write letters or make phone calls to your local legislators. Consider providing testimony at committee hearings on proposed bills. Who knows better than a healthcare worker what patients' needs are?

As healthcare workers you must become active participants in the legislative process. Influencing and changing the future of healthcare by educating lawmakers can make a difference. The need for grassroots support and advocacy has never been more important. You must contribute time and energy to the legislative process at a grassroots level in order to exert control over your destiny.

Discussion Questions:

1. Define professional advocacy and explain why it is important.
2. Explain ways to be a professional advocate.
3. List characteristics of remarkable employees.
4. Explain who is responsible for healthcare worker retention and why.
5. Discuss retention strategies for healthcare workers in your specialty and why they might be effective.
6. Identify key survival strategies during turbulent times.
7. List 3 risks and 3 rewards for using survival strategies
8. Explain the concept of networking and why it is important
9. List 5 activities that are part of networking
10. Explain the purpose and value of joining a professional organization.
11. Discuss the value of political advocacy.

Case Study:

1. Use Yahoo CEO case study to discuss embellishment vs. integrity, risks and rewards of both

http://articles.latimes.com/2012/may/14/business/la-fi-yahoo-thompson-resigns-20120514

SUPERVISION AND
MANAGEMENT OF WORKERS

PORTRAIT OF A LEADER

- Persistence. Not insistence. A strong leader hangs on a little longer, works a little harder.
- Imagination. S/he harnesses imagination to practical plans that produce results.
- Vision. The present is just the beginning. A good leader is impressed with the possibilities of the future.
- Sincerity. A good leader can be trusted.
- Integrity. A good leader has principles and lives by them.
- Poise. A good leader is not overbearing, but friendly and assured.
- Thoughtfulness. S/he is considerate and aware.
- Common Sense. A good leader has good judgment based on reason
- Altruism. A good leader lives by the Golden Rule.
- Initiative. S/he gets things started now!

Author unknown

SUPERVISION AND MANAGEMENT

Chapter Objectives:

1. Define the role of a supervisor
2. Explain the difference between authoritarian and participative management styles.
3. Discuss the concept of discipline.
4. List 6 unforgivable supervisory mistakes.
5. Explain the different management theories including theory X,Y,Z,C,T
6. Identify 6 differences between managers and leaders.
7. Explain the process of decision making
8. Explain the process of problem solving

Key terms

Supervision	Management techniques	Delegation
Power	Influence	
Management	Discipline	
Leadership	Decision making	
Problem solving	Management theories	

Supervising the work of others

A supervisor, more than anything else, is a leader. The supervisor accomplishes tasks through other people so that the organization's goals can be achieved. The supervisor sets the tempo, guides people's efforts, provides inspiration, and sometimes nudges people along, while at other times exercises discipline and delivers constructive criticism. Supervision is a constant balancing act of trying to keep a positive team spirit alive in the department or work unit. Supervision means setting goals and guiding staff towards them.

Some supervisors appear to have natural leadership ability, but most supervisors have had to develop their skills through experience and training. Different management techniques have been identified, but generally there are two kinds of management philosophy. They are authoritarian and participative. Authoritarian management involves rigidly defined individual responsibility as a means of avoiding confusion as to who does what. It tends to foster competition among the members of a work unit. Generally, authoritarian management involves the assumption that people are passive, lack ambition are indifferent to organizational needs and need to be controlled. Essential tasks of authoritarian based supervisors are to direct, control and motivate others.

Participative supervisors understand that responsibility is more flexible since it is clarified through discussion and group consensus. Participative styles tend to foster cooperation and teamwork among the members of a work unit. It involves the assumption that people have the motivation, the potential development, and the readiness to direct behavior toward organizational goals. Essential tasks of participative supervisors are to arrange organizational conditions and methods of operation in such a way that people can achieve their own goals best by directing their efforts toward organizational objectives.

It wasn't all that long ago that many supervisors in this country believed in and practices an authoritarian management style. It became very clear that the authoritarian approach did not promote employee participation in the work processes. The people performing the essential tasks of providing the services or producing the products were not involved in the workplace decisions that directly impacted the quality of the services or products. Because of this, management and supervisors were uninformed about problems or opportunities for improvement in the work processes which then resulted in poor product quality and services.

After World War II, the Japanese adopted a management philosophy which was more participative in design. It was important that they do this as their country needed to be rebuilt after the war. They focused on continuous quality improvement and included employees in the work processes which enhanced quality and results. Because the Japanese were more responsive to customers' needs, they have captured markets, such as the automotive markets away from the US. This management style promotes quality and employee participation in the work processes and decisions.

In the mid twentieth century, many American companies starting using the participative management style. They now believe in the importance of ensuring employee participation is built into work processes, so that quality products and services can be the standard outcome. This type of management philosophy has had proven results. The automobile and airline industries have adopted and revised this strategy and have increased their markets from foreign competitors.

There is a time to apply the authoritarian management style and use it successfully. Some workplace decisions require quick decisiveness on the part of management where consensus and participation are not practical and should not be applied. Disasters and code blues are good examples of this in healthcare settings. In reality, most successful managers and supervisors know when to use participative leadership skills and when it is necessary to utilize an authoritarian approach, or a blend of both philosophies. There is a continuum of management styles that are recommended based on the urgency and complexity of the decision, level of employee expertise and the extent of the parameters when making the decision.

To be effective, supervisors must have priorities on what to do. As a supervisor, one of the most important tasks is that of teaching and training. When a new person comes on the job, it is the supervisor's responsibility to see to it that they know what they are doing before they are assigned a task to perform. If you simply assume that they can do the job, you may find yourself in lots of trouble.

Training responsibility involves more than instructing new staff. It is important to keep informed about new developments and information and pass that along to your staff. Whenever a new method of doing something or a new regulation is introduced, the supervisor must see to it that staff has the skills necessary to perform those procedures. Supervisors are also responsible for safety on the unit. Safety not only applies to all people in the facility, but to any equipment used as well. By setting a good example and applying the rules to everyone, the supervisor assures that the facility safety regulations will be followed exactly.

Perhaps the most difficult responsibility of a supervisor is discipline. Authoritarian managers often use threats and abusive language as discipline. This method is ineffective because it causes fear and resentment in staff that slows down work and makes people feel uncooperative. A successful supervisor attempts to discipline using the positive approach. Positive discipline means that the person being disciplined should realize that the discipline is to help them do a better job and not to punish or embarrass them.

Positive discipline can be achieved by following these principles:

- Discipline should be handled professionally and impersonally; not as an attack on the individual

- Discipline should be applied as soon as the situation will allow (but not when the supervisor is angry)

- Discipline should always be applied to everyone in the same way=fairly

- Staff members must be informed of rules and regulations in advance.

Both constructive criticism and discipline should be handled privately and confidentially with only the individual. Certain exceptions apply if the facility is unionized and union representatives can be involved. Handling discipline on an impersonal basis means that the discipline is directed against a behavior or violation, not against the person. A person is not punished because they failed to follow a safety regulation. They are shown the serious consequences that could result from not complying with a rule designed to make their job (and the patient) a safer one.

It is also important for a supervisor to have a positive attitude. This is frequently not emphasized in training, but it is crucial for success. When a supervisor is positive, productivity improves. When a supervisor is negative, productivity drops. The challenge is to remain positive, even if those around you are not.

People are all motivated by essentially the same things. Accomplishments, recognition, new challenges and learning new things are the same basic needs for all people. Supervisors should strive to create the environment that fosters employees to achieve and be motivated themselves.

 **For your toolkit... Six Unforgivable Supervisory Mistakes**

1. **Treating individuals unequally because of sex, culture, age, disability, etc. Besides being illegal, every employee deserves the same consideration.**

2. **Not keeping your word. The fastest way to destroy a trusting relationship with a subordinate is to make a promise and then break it.**

3. **Blowing hot and cold. Consistency is essential when managing. If you are positive one day and negative the next, staff will not know how to react. Respect for you will disappear.**

4. **Failure to follow basic company/facility policies and procedures. As a supervisor, you must handle your relationship with each staff member in a consistent and legal manner. This means doing things like documenting clarification of expectations and employee improvement plans before telling a manager you wish to terminate an employee.**

5. **Losing your cool in front of staff. Everyone reaches their threshold of tolerance on occasion, but you need to keep your temper in check and your emotions under control. Blowing up can destroy relationships.**

6. **Engaging in a personal relationship with someone you supervise. No matter how close you are to staff members when you are both staff; when you are a supervisor, you change your role. It is poor practice to be in charge of a person during the day and personally involved with that individual after work.**

Successful/unsuccessful supervisory traits

Successful supervisors	Unsuccessful supervisors
Remain positive under stress	Permit problems to get to them
Take time to teach what they know	Rush instructions to staff, then fail to follow-up
Build/maintain rewarding relationships with subordinates	Insensitive to subordinates needs
Learn to set reasonable and consistent lines of authority	Not interested in learning supervisory skills
Learn to delegate	Fail to understand that it isn't what a supervisor can do, but what they can get others to accomplish
Establish standards of high quality and set good examples	Let their status go to their head
Work hard to become good communicators	Continue to offer one way communication
Build team efforts to achieve high productivity	Become too authoritarian or too lax

Supervisors have specific responsibilities in accordance with the overall business of a healthcare facility. As a supervisor, your responsibility is to manage your responsibilities as part of the overall business. You are responsible for the proper and efficient use of people, equipment and resources to run a smooth operation. Efficient use of people and supplies means controlling your job so that these resources are not wasted. Your efforts to get the job done correctly, efficiently, and on time are essential to the success of the facility.

Your relationship with patients is also very important in maintaining their satisfaction with the facility and care. If there is a delay, explain what is happening. If the patient has specific expectations about their care, do your best to see that they are done that way, without violating facility policies, regulations or safety standards. A good supervisor is essentially a salesperson selling your healthcare facility to the patients. There have been many times when a supervisor and staff do a great technical job with care, but offended a patient in the process. The result was that the facility lost future business. On the other hand, if a job goes poorly, a good supervisor who relates well with patients can still project a good facility image. Good customer relations are important because they can develop goodwill and contribute to the growth of the facility.

Another responsibility you have as a supervisor is to your staff members. You need to make sure that each person is working in a job they are best suited to handle. Training and education can help each person become more qualified and more productive. You are responsible for assigning daily tasks so that each staff member on your team knows what they are expected to do and when and how they are expected to do it.

You must ensure that each person has the necessary tools, equipment and materials to safely complete their assigned job tasks. As a supervisor, you relay company policy to your staff. You have an obligation to present management directives to your staff as if they were your own. This is true even if you do not always completely agree with them. You are the linchpin between your staff members and upper management. Successful supervisors can quickly gain the respect and confidence of a work unit by showing staff that the supervisor will present their opinions to upper management and stand by them.

Successful supervisors know their people and realize that they have individual differences. You can learn about each person as an individual by listening to them and observing their actions. You must be a problem solver and let staff know they can come to you with their concerns. Be aware that every staff member has personal problems away from the job that may affect their performance. In your supervisory role, you must be alert to these problems and be willing to help resolve (or refer) them as well as job related problems.

Supervisors cannot motivate their employees alone. But they are essential in creating the organizational climate that motivates employees to perform their jobs effectively. Not only does the supervisor need to create the work environment that allows staff members to self-motivate, but they also need to look at their own behaviors and traits to ensure employees feel respected and valued as a member of the work team.

Effective supervision includes:

- Being organized so you have more time for goal setting and dealing with subordinates
- Delegate effectively
- Communicate effectively
- Discipline appropriately

Supervisors that Delegate effectively:

- Explain importance of job
- Explain end results and let the employee determine how the task will e completed
- Clearly define the employee's authority and/or parameters that the employee has when completing the task
- Agree on a deadline and time frame with the employee
- Ask for feedback to ensure the employee completely understands the tasks and your expectations
- Provide controls to ensure the employee is on the right track. Follow-up and check on the employee's progress on the task.

Supervisors that communicate effectively:

- Plan for the communication with the employee. Schedule a time and plan what you want to say.
- Be honest, candid, specific and factual. Provide examples
- Open up communication with open ended questions. Remember to listen, as it needs to be two way communication
- Ask for feedback. Ensure that you and the employee have a shared understanding of the goal. Everyone has the need to feel important enough to be asked for their views.

Supervisors that discipline appropriately:

- Give facts and figures unemotionally
- Help the employee understand why s/he is being disciplined, and define the problem.
- Get agreement that a problem exists
- Look for solutions to resolve the performance problem/conduct

What skills are required in a Charge Role?

Most healthcare facilities have someone in charge of each unit or shift. Most often they are called Lead, Charge, or Shift Supervisor. Whatever the title, the role includes direct accountability for one unit on one shift. This is the first step in becoming a supervisor and usually a step before becoming a manager.

Outstanding charge personnel are easy to spot. They have the following characteristics:

- Support a successful quality improvement program
- Achieving JCAHO accreditation with no contingencies
- Controlling total labor cost per patient day
- Controlling contract (registry/travelers) per patient day
- Achieving outstanding physician satisfaction survey results
- Achieving outstanding patient satisfaction survey results
- Supporting new program implementation
- Maintaining costs per unit within 5% of budget

The charge personnel of the past were different than those that are needed today. The "old mental model" of charge staff included difficult mentalities such as; the world is fair or there is a shortage and that's it. Charge staff acted as if contract labor (registry and travelers) was inevitable, and that a licensed caregiver-only model is best for patient care even if it isn't practical in today's environment. Healthcare salaries were perceived as pitifully poor and therefore it was assumed productivity cannot be enhanced. It was assumed that all healthcare staff is professionally motivated and would do things just because they needed doing. This mentality no longer has a place in healthcare.

The "new charge personnel model" is based on delivering quality and effective care at a lower costs, using staff in differentiated roles based on education and training, working in a team model, focusing on high levels of patient, physician and family satisfaction, eliminating things for staff to do that don't make a difference, being creative and innovative when solving problems, managing limited resources and adopting a customer focused orientation about healthcare.

Successful charge personnel in this century need to focus on using less management staff to support their decisions, identifying who is the coordinator of care, eliminating duplication, cross training whenever possible, eliminating barriers between departments, and eliminating non-productive time. They also set standards for quality and customer service measures, rewards and sanctions. Charge personnel help with decentralizing recruitment/retention, education, QA, UR, infection control and risk management as every unit's accountability and responsibility. Charge people experience an increased use of technology, staff by cost and unit of service not only acuity, become more customer sensitive by moving services to the customer, and streamline documentation.

The ability to communicate well with staff is crucial. Lack of communication by managers is one of several key reasons leading to conflicts with staff members in healthcare settings today according to several studies. Good communication skills are vital to developing a happy productive staff willing to do more when crises arise. Because healthcare managers often move between multiple units and balance their time between each unit, it is a challenge for managers to be available to staff. Therefore, the charge person becomes the available spokesperson for the manager. This helps to support staff and maintain patient care quality and satisfaction. Charge personnel end up managing day to day operations on a specific unit because the manager is overseeing day to day operations on multiple units, plus assuring quality patient care, patient safety, staff development and education, staff satisfaction, recruitment, retention, financial analysis and multidisciplinary meetings and teams.

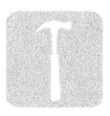

For your toolkit... Lack of communication by healthcare managers is a key reason for conflict with staff members

The charge personnel become a crucial conduit for the healthcare manager with staff on a unit. Open communication and candid conversations go a long way to preventing unresolved conflict. If there is an issue, talking about it is essential. Having good dialog with staff and listening responsively to individuals is also important, and charge personnel can provide that conduit as well. This creates mutual respect and collaboration, which improves both patient care and staff morale. Charge personnel are essential ingredients to making that happen effectively on a unit.

Mentoring and support for new charge personnel, as well as resources and training are crucial to their success. Charge personnel need to be selected on their ability to supervise the work of others, not just because they are good clinicians. Charge personnel support their healthcare manager with key functions. The healthcare manager role is probably the most difficult role in healthcare. I always felt like I was stuck between the staff and administration. I had 24 hour accountability, and without my charge personnel, I could never have made it work.

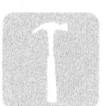

For your toolkit... Being a manager is the most challenging role in healthcare.

Key experience and attributes of charge personnel in today's healthcare industry include:

1. Education/experience

- Specialty license e.g. pharmacist, radiology technologist, registered nurse
- Three to four years experience as a staff member with shift/team accountability
- Bachelors' degree completed or in progress

2. Technical Expertise

- Understanding JCAHO accreditation and regulatory requirements for your specialty and the facility
- Understanding of cost per unit standards
- Staff supervision and oversight
- Strong ability to plan and coordinate staff and unit activity

3. Basic Skills

- Leadership
- Delegation
- Directing
- Motivating
- Supervising the work of others
- Organizational skills
- Critical thinking skills
- Sound judgment

4. Decision making ability
5. Integrity
6. Objective perspective/independent thinker
7. Strong work ethic/high energy level
8. Good time management skills
9. Strong and positive self image
10. Effective interpersonal skills
11. Flexible/adaptable and excited by change
12. Assertiveness and tenacity
13. Drive and personal ambition
14. Self motivated/self starter

Competency Profile for Outstanding Charge Personnel

Achievement competencies:

- Drive for achievement
- Initiative
- Concern for order

Influence competencies:

- Interpersonal sensitivity
- Awareness and concern of personal impact
- Direct persuasion
- Use of influence strategies
- Organizational awareness
- Relationship building

Self Management competencies:

- Self-confidence
- Tenacity
- Self-control
- Flexibility

Problem solving competencies:

- Use of concepts
- Analytical thinking
- Pattern recognition
- Technical expertise

Managerial competencies:

- Development of others
- Directing others
- Management of groups
- Efficiency orientation
- Motivation of others
- Cause/effect thinking
- Creativity and innovation
- Calculated risk taking
- Concern with image and impact
- Empathy

Knowledge/qualifications

- Bachelor's degree
- Business appreciation

Social/communication skills

- Fluent verbal skills
- Good listening skills
- Developing presentation skills
- Developing negotiation skills
- Positive self presentation
- Rapport building
- Social deportment
- Cooperativeness
- Ability to inspire others

Personal Traits

- Enthusiasm
- Decisiveness
- Stress tolerance
- Self-motivation
- Tolerance for ambiguity

*Adapted from "Traits of an Indispensable Nurse" lecture by Richard B. Brock, RN, BA, BSN, MA, NEA-BC
Care Experience Coordinator Nursing, Kaiser Permanente Los Angeles Medical Center

Analyze your leadership strengths and weaknesses. There are several leadership theories that have been outlined in the business world over the past several decades. In a nutshell these are:

Leadership Theory	Driving thought
Theory X	No one really wants to work
Theory Y	Individuals really want to make a contribution
Theory Z	People work best in teams
Theory C	If you satisfy the customer, you will have a future
Transformational leadership theory	Visionary, risk taker, confidence builder, and change artist

In "Peanut Butter and Jelly Management: Tales from Parenthood Lessons for Managers" (Amacom, 2004), the Komisarjevskys detail how being a good manager, or demonstrating your capability to be a good manager, requires many of the same skills as being a good parent.

Some say that leaders are born, not made. William A. Cohen, Ph.D., retired major general of the U.S. Air Force, would beg to differ.

"Leadership can be learned," he says. "It's a matter of not only having the qualities [of a leader], but knowing what to do." (2004) Even if you're a long shot for a promotion at work, ask the bosses to consider you it will show you're ambitious and anxious for more responsibility. Or suggest creating a task force to temporarily fill the void left by the open position. You boss will not only be impressed by your ambition, but your desire to lead as well.

These are the difference between managers and leaders:

Managers	Leaders
Do things right	Do the right things
Solve problems	Avoid problems
Follow direction	Obtain results
Manage productivity	Increase profits
Are efficient	Are effective
Maintain compliance	Improve the system
Control	Influence
Work in hierarchy	Work in network
Make plans	Enhance learning
Create transaction	Create transformation
Administers	Innovates
Copies	Starts from original
Maintains	Develops
Focuses on systems and structure	Focuses on people
Relies on control	Inspires trust
Uses short range viewpoint	Uses long range perspective
Keeps eyes on bottom line	Has eyes on the horizon
Asks how and when	Asks what and why
Accepts the status quo	Challenges status quo
Classic good soldier	Own individual person

Leaders for professional staff are like yeast is to bread or fuel is to a rocket. You can't have one without the other. Managers and charge personnel need subordinates more than subordinates need them. Managers get paid for what the subordinates do and create–not only for what they do themselves. Charge personnel need to have:

- Supervisory skills
- Ability to respond to ambiguity and rapid change
- Ability to manage self as well as others
- Ability to communicate organizations vision to employees
- Excellent time management skills
- Positive, professional role model
- Ability to develop trust in employees
- Ability to foster innovation in employees
- Ability to maintain perspective and sense of humor

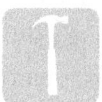 **For your toolkit... Leaders for professional staff are like yeast is to bread or fuel is to a rocket. You can't have one without the other.**

Charge personnel core competencies include:

- Problem solving
- Management
- Influence
- Social and communication skills
- Achievement
- Self-management
- Keeps external focus
- Promotes vision and values for the future
- Promotes continual quality and process improvement
- Acts as a change agent
- Values people
- Demonstrates skills of management especially under circumstances of uncertainty or conflict
- Decentralizes information and authority
- Pursues self development

Should You Be A Healthcare Manager?

Managers are paid to make tough decisions. They must make trade-offs in how resources are distributed, balance different interests in complex and ambiguous situations and use their clout to defined their units interests without undermining the performance of the entire organization. (2008) Managers need power to do this type of work, but many think that the primary power source comes from their formal authority. What is required to do the job well is not just being in control, but gaining the support and commitment of subordinates, peers and higher-ups as collaborators. Formal authority can often effect changes in behavior, but for commitment or changes in attitude, managers have to share their power with subordinates.

The idea of empowerment makes one think of losing control; however, sharing power with others actually increases a manager's influence in a situation. This is the paradox of power. Empowerment means sharing the potential to influence others. By granting others the autonomy to do their jobs, and sharing information and expertise to ensure they make sound judgment calls, managers hold great influence over workers. The manager still sets the agenda within which work should be accomplished, but those closest to the action can figure out tactics and solve problems.

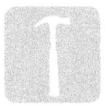 **For your toolkit… Sharing power with others actually increases a manager's influence.**

It gets a bit stickier when a manager must influence those over whom s/he has no direct or formal authority. In order to influence folks over which you have no authority, you need allies. Peers as well as higher ups are sources of critical information, resources and collaboration. By setting up a network with these folks, a manager creates allies. When a manager creates allies, s/he enhances her/his influence as well as the ability to get the job done.

Smart managers regard anyone they depend on as a potential ally, even if the individual appears to be an adversary. The focus is on building mutually beneficial alliances by discerning what the manager can offer that allies may need or want. In order to exercise influence through exchange, you must first identify those on whom you are dependent, and then step into their shoes to see the world from their perspective. In order to use this strategy, you must know who you are dependent on and why, whose cooperation and compliance are needed and whose opposition will keep you from accomplishing your work. Your source of power becomes what you have to offer that they need or want, and what they have to offer that you need or want. Trust will drive your source of power. Mutual trust will allow you to build influence.

When assessing relationships and making sense of situations in which there are perceived conflicts of interest, it is likely that managers determine their own behavior as honorable, and that of the other person as self-aggrandizing, irrational or ambitious. It is important to not attribute malicious motives to those opposing you in a conflict situation. It is important for you to test your assumptions and adopt a broader perspective–this is crucial for win-win negotiations.

Ensuring you have a network that includes relationships with many different people is hard work, but worthwhile. It is how you can be successful as a manager. Since most of us are most comfortable with those similar to us, the larger challenge lies in bridging differences. Concentrate on people who are critical to success, but with whom you do not have a well developed relationship.

Trust is a function of how an individual perceives a manager in three areas. These area are competence (does s/he know the right thing to do?), character (does s/he want to do the right thing?) and influence (can s/he get it done?). The more trust people have in you, the less often they will require "proof" that you will deliver what you have promised. This kind of flexibility is invaluable to managers, especially during organizational upheavals.

Thinking about influence as an exchange can lead some managers to be exploitive. Remember, to work, networks have to be mutually beneficial. Treating people fairly is to treat them differently–based on what *they* need. Exercising influence depends on being clear about that. Be aware of not only achieving your immediate objective, but also on how your actions will affect a relationship over time. Influence is about building interdependencies, and creating partnerships is one of the most rewarding aspects of management.

Responsibilities of managers in leadership roles

Be the source of a vision
Establish and maintain trust
Serve as a political conduit
Serve as ethical standard bearer for the unit/department
Make decisions
Make effective and appropriate judgments
Expand awareness of staff
Become a spark
Build a framework for effective communication
Adopt a constant planning perspective and attitude

Being a manager can be one of the most rewarding career moves a healthcare worker can make. It can also be the most frustrating. Being a manager involves being a leader, as well as supervising the work of others. You are both the drum major leading the parade and the band master pushing from the rear of the band to keep things moving. I have been in about eight different types of management roles in my career. I have learned much about how to manage in thirty six years in nursing–both from doing it right *and* doing it wrong. If you are considering moving into management and move into the healthcare administration arena, there are some issues you need to evaluate.

Are you willing to get additional training? Expanding your job-related education is an effective way to move ahead. Obtaining an academic degree isn't always necessary, but acquiring essential management skills sets definitely is. Employers are looking for excellent written and oral communication, and an ability to effectively manage staff and workloads. If you are interested in a management promotion, consider taking classes that focus on supervision and communication skills. There are national programs that offer one-day seminars, local college and online course options.

Are you able to coach others? The ability to motivate others and oversee their work is critical in most healthcare roles, but particularly in management. If you are a computer whiz, offer to train co-workers, even if it is not part of your present job description. This will provide supervisory experience beyond the scope of your job. Whenever possible, volunteer to oversee per diem or registry staff, or head up a committee or project. These activities will make sure you know how to give clear directions and to tactfully check to see that the work is progressing correctly and in a timely manner. Evaluate your awareness that there are multiple ways to get a job done effectively, and a job can be well done—even if it isn't done the way you would do it. The art of coaching is discussed in depth in the Coaching/ mentoring chapter.

Can you make decisions and delegate? Both are key functions of managers. If you are a parent or care for a dependent, you likely already do both skills well. Managers must assign tasks, plan projects, and make numerous choices daily. Practice implementing these skills on your job, at home or in community activities. Become active in professional healthcare organizations and take on leadership roles. Learn how to give assignments to others, taking care to provide the time and resources necessary to help them complete the tasks at hand.

Do you have the initiative and willingness to take on responsibility? Managers must be able to operate independently and be self-directed. They must be able to make significant contributions to productivity and the financial bottom line of a facility. With more regulations, shorter lengths of stay and higher patient acuity, managers have to work faster and smarter just to stay up with the workload. Make it a habit to ask for more work and expand the scope of your current job. This will help you get used to the frequent requests from your boss to "take a look at this situation and give me your recommendations" that comes with being a manager. Contribute new ideas to management for ways to improve your department or unit.

Do you have strong communication skills? The ability to listen, explain clearly and give precise directions is crucial. Oral and written skills are paramount in management success, but communicating effectively also means using technology to transmit information. Practice speaking at and facilitating meetings. Volunteer to serve on department committees and be an active participant. Improve your written skills by writing reports or correspondence.

Are you a good listener? Listening is a critical part of communication, and is covered in the chapter on communication skills. Employers want managers who ask for and listen to ideas and suggestions. Pay close attention as colleagues' state their requests or outline a problem. Be conscious of letting a person explain while you take in what is being said. Do not interrupt. Managers, however hurried or pressured they may be, need to allow others to express themselves completely, whenever possible. Once you have heard everything, formulate your response. This way, both employers and those you supervise will view interactions with you in a positive way.

Have you studied other managers? Observe managers you respect and those you don't respect and analyze their skills. How assertive are they? How do they make decisions? Are they polite and respectful of employees and subordinates? Do they listen? Do they accept feedback graciously? Do they follow up with employee issues? Emulate their strengths to develop your own style. Learn how to handle problems by watching what managers do well or not so well. You can also learn a lot by watching someone who is an ineffective manager. Learning how *not* to behave can be as valuable as a positive role model. Seek advice on how to motivate others and manage workload. People work hardest for and are most loyal to managers who praise and reward good work.

Do you use professional ethics? Managers must display high moral standards. Do you respect other employees? Are you careful not to offend other staff? Are you sensitive to diversity issues? Are you careful not to use terminology that others might deem offensive? Do you treat all people fairly? In today's healthcare environment, it is especially important to show a high level of integrity and avoid actions that could be seen as discriminatory or harassing or that demonstrate a different care standard for patients.

Can you handle deadlines as well as set and meet goals? The higher in an organization you move, the more pressure you will encounter, so you need to develop coping mechanisms that will help you handle challenges without burning out. Good time management skills and organizing your work efficiently are essential. When you plan projects, develop a timeline that outlines the tasks. As your workload and the number of staff under you increase, you will need to become extremely well organized. You need to create a foundation to deal effectively with problems as they arise.

Another essential skill for leadership is observation. Notice who the leaders are. True leaders are individuals whom people gravitate to. Using a true leader as a mentor offers valuable insight into your behavior, as well as discussing what works and what doesn't with an expert. Keep in mind that not all mentoring experiences are positive. I have learned a lot about how *not* to behave by watching some leaders in nursing and healthcare.

Leaders actually lead by effective communication, empowering followers, having a clear vision, seeing he bigger picture, navigating around potential pitfalls and have positive self confidence. Leaders tend to fail when success goes to their head, they establish a personal kingdom, and misled into believing they are infallible and need no one else. One way to keep egos in check is to realize that leaders wouldn't have a role to lead without people to lead. Therefore, a crucial duty is to empower your followers by creating a sense of significance, competence and community. Keeping open lines of honest communication and showing employees how their work contributes to a meaningful end is a great way to create an all-inclusive environment for success.

When evaluating one's potential as a manager, there are a few areas to consider, such as decision-making strategies, problem solving skills, self confidence, interpersonal skills, facilitation, adaptability, integrity, commitment and empathy. Assessing your own strengths and weaknesses will allow you to see where your skills are developmentally at the present time. This requires honesty about the raw materials you have to work with. Evaluating where you are will help you determine what you hope to become as a manager.

Can you do all the things just listed? Then a management role could be next up for you. Now that you are willing to consider a management position, there are some additional things you need to know. First and foremost, if you are going to lead, lead well. There are plenty of lousy healthcare managers. We don't need more of those. We have all worked with toxic managers and it is extremely demoralizing. Effective, positive managers are also linked to staff retention. All the best recruitment strategies are for naught if staff members leave due to a toxic manager.

As a new manager, you will want to create a few strategies to enhance your chance of success. Here are some strategies I have used effectively when starting in a new management role. Open your office door and be available and visible. Staff isn't sure what you are up to if they can't see you. Be seen. Hanging out with staff at planned meetings, lunches and breaks works very well. You can learn more about what is happening on your unit by hanging around the coffee pot than you ever will in a meeting. Be honest and deal with staff fears like system changes, reductions in force or staff shortages. Staff may not talk about what they are really worried about when you are new, so you need to talk about what you think people are really thinking and feelings. When fears are mentioned out in the open and discussed, you can create trust and establish a relationship.

Don't fall into the common trap of assuming people will know how to act if you are their manager. Many managers assume that subordinates will read minds to understand what the manager wants in terms of outcomes and behavior. Some managers believe that if people are smart enough, they will just figure out what you want. Nothing is further from the truth. Staff needs to be clear on your expectations and understand your style. It's great if employees can read the subtle nuances in your behavior and figure out exactly what you require of them.

But most people aren't mind readers. Even those that are smart may be oblivious to what's important to you unless you spell it out. If you have the CEO of the hospital visit your department, some of your employees will naturally put "their best foot forward" and do a good job of demonstrating that "Everything is fine here!" but many will use that opportunity to explain problems and frustrations. If you want those employees to behave differently, you will need to explain how you want them to behave when an administrator comes on the unit.

In most hospital departments, if employees ask for information, they get it, but most managers would prefer that certain kinds of information be withheld or "glossed over" with a VIP on the unit. It may seem that you really should not to ask people to do what they have to do to make the department, the hospital, them —and you— look good. It's not that these things are immoral. It's just that they lie outside of what we consider usual job requirements. People are often given incomplete or incorrect information and expected to know exactly what to use and what to disregard. Twenty percent of your staff will know. The other eighty percent will be confused, frustrated and ultimately inefficient.

Counting on your employees to read minds is an all-too-common management style that often results in disappointment and distrust. Managers feel impatient and irritated with employees who need more specific information. Employees sense that they have disappointed the boss but usually have no idea what they need to do to meet expectations. After all, they are not mind readers.

All skills and abilities are distributed along a normal curve. This means that 20% percent of any group will be superior performers, 60% will be average, and 20% below average (Robbins, 2009). Some folks are at the top end of the normal curve for observational learning. This is the learning people do by watching successful people and imitating what they do.

Studies show that about 20% of any group of employees will be good enough at learning by observation to figure out what it is expected (2009). Those employees need minimal direction and little support. Bosses often see these top performers and wonder why the rest of their employees can't figure out what it takes. They expect the same behaviors and abilities from the other 80 percent and both sides end up frustrated.

Intelligent people often assume that everybody else knows as much as they know and can do what they do. They might think of people who can't do what they do as stupid, but more often they will see them as lacking motivation. When we know something, it seems so obvious that we forget how it felt not to know it. To others, however, who don't know exactly what we know in the way that we know it, we seem to expect them to be mind readers. The illusion is that getting better at our jobs means building up an ever-enlarging collection of facts. The facts come early in the learning process. Increases in skill don't come from an increase in the store of facts in your head, but rather in the ability to make finer and finer distinctions.

Most managers can be good at doing, but may not be skilled at analyzing what they do and explaining it to other people. They may also assume that explaining is what teachers do. In reality, the best managers have skills of good teachers. Teachers assume that students don't know what the teacher knows, and that the main purpose of teaching is to get them to understand the subject as well as the teacher does. Too many managers think that employees already know whatever they need to know. Nothing is further from the truth.

One of the real tests of your skills as a manager is the effect you have on the majority of people who don't know what you want intuitively. These people are paying attention to some cues, but those cues may not be the ones you want them to follow. The more you really manage, the more effective you will be and the less mind reading will be required.

Decide what you want your staff to know. Before you teach them, understand exactly what you want your staff to learn. Let them know in advance what they are supposed to do, when to do it, and how they can meet your expectations. Ask for what you want and don't assume that people know what to do. Most people know the basics of the job. What you need them to learn specifically is matters of style and the manner in which things are done on your unit. They must also understand and be sensitive to the political realities in your facility. It's probably best to assume that the people you manage know absolutely nothing about these kinds of things except what you tell them. Set priorities and tell people what they are. Break complex skills into parts when you explain them. Use examples that apply to your unit. Encourage questions as you teach.

Reward good work and that behavior will happen more often. Usually the strategy of managers is to do the opposite. As long as employees are doing what they are supposed to be doing, they are often ignored. Then, when they step out of line, they are punished. Punishing negative behavior is much less effective than rewarding positive behavior. The more pay off there is for doing what you want; the more likely you are to get it.

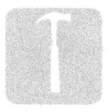 **For your toolkit... Reward good work and that behavior will happen more often.**

It is difficult to instill attitudes that lead to correct behavior. Make a practical detailed request and even show people what you want if you can. Tell them why they should do it. You don't need to worry what they are thinking while they are doing what you want. That will come with time, as they gain experience.

You will also need to talk to your employees. Ask about and listen to their concerns. Ask questions to determine their understanding of how things really are. The better you know them, the better you will know what they need to know. Short, regular meetings for exactly this purpose are helpful. The more you can get your employees to talk to you, the more effective you can be as their boss.

You will need to tell them explicitly what is to be done in certain situations. Tell it like it is, even if you are embarrassed. Give them examples of what is appropriate or inappropriate, even if the examples are difficult or embarrassing for you. You will be much more embarrassed if the people you oversee don't know these things.

Be sure you deal with conflict. Groups of people and team members will invariably experience conflict. Many managers choose to ignore conflict when new to a role and hope that it will go away. Some choose to use coercion to get staff to change. As many of us have experienced, this doesn't work well in healthcare (or anywhere else for that matter). To deal with conflict among your staff, start by asking those who disagree to paraphrase one another's comments. This may help them learn whether they really understand each other. Work out a compromise. Agree on the underlying source of conflict and then engage in give-and take- discussions to finally agree on a solution. Ask each person to list what the others should do. Exchange lists and select a compromise that all are willing to accept-even if they don't like it.

You may need to convince some team members that they have to admit they were incorrect. Help them save face by convincing them that changing a position may actually show strength and assertive maturity. Last but not least, respect the experts on your team. Give their opinions more weight when the conflict involves their expertise, but don't rule out conflicting opinions. Creative conflict resolution can be positive for everyone involved.

Be sure you share information. Staff need to know what upper management is thinking and planning. If staff feels uninformed, they perceive changes are being "done to them" instead of feeling they are involved in making the changes. That is why it is so effective to use "pot stirrers" as project coordinators. It puts all that energy to positive use! Use newsletters, email memos, and regular meetings to keep staff up to date. Involve your employees. Ask staff for input and ideas on how to improve services or enhance systems. Reward innovators and follow up on suggestions.

Remember to give it time. It takes time for new managers to learn how to be effective. It takes time for staff to trust and respect new managers. Be patient, and remember you cannot rush the process of learning how to be a good manager. Research studies identify retention strategies related to the work environment as critical to employee satisfaction. 50% of employee satisfaction comes from their relationship with their bosses. (Kaye, 2002) Research shows that the quality of the relationship between a boss and subordinate is a primary predictor of intentions to remain in a current workplace.

An investment in strengthening an organization's leaders– from senior executives to middle managers to team leaders– pays off in all sorts of ways, but particularly in attracting and retaining employees. Healthcare managers have a responsibility to learn how to manage proactively and effectively. This benefits not only their individual life long learning, but their employees' well being and satisfaction with the organization.

Those hospitals that have measures in place to hold managers accountable for retention tended to experience lower turnover rates. Accountability measures can include incorporation of retention efforts into the managers' performance appraisal process, bonuses for taking action related to turnover or achieving a qualitative or quantitative change in the turnover rate, and periodic review of employee satisfaction in the manager's specific service area. (Abrahms, 2002)

Risks of being a manager	Rewards of being a manager
Inability to be positive 100% of time	Empowerment
Increased stress	Increased self confidence
Lack of security	Expanding horizons
Feel "caught in the middle"	Personal growth
Crises orientated basis of function	Satisfaction from helping others grow
Changing relationships	Building professionalism/pride
Failure	Success
"Doesn't feel fun anymore"	Feel passionate and excited about work

Focusing on retention strategies means facilities cannot ignore the effect that leadership style has on retention. Toxic healthcare executives and middle managers can sabotage retention efforts by driving away staff at all levels of the organization. The best retention strategies in the world will not work if retention is inhibited by self-centered, power-hungry leaders.

Healthcare staff will both be wary of executives and managers who impede retention by setting up a personal kingdom instead of working as a team, using fear and intimidation to get tasks completed, a "my way or the highway" mentality, making negative comments about staff, or blaming subordinates for decisions that result in poor outcomes. Healthcare staff who work under retention-inhibiting conditions often complain about their work environment and change positions. Toxic attitudes can spread outward and cause a ripple affect that can damage an entire facility and take years to repair.

A positive leadership style is a cornerstone of success as well as a key retention strategy. Healthcare leaders who reward efforts with positive feedback, encouragement and coaching are also retaining staff. Career enhancement as well as retention-focused behaviors include empowerment of staff at all levels, coaching for both positive change and to eliminate negative behaviors, choosing to mentor both new staff and new managers, investment in training and skill building for all levels of staff, implementing change with a teamwork-based model, encouraging innovation and out-of-the-box thinking for care management and work redesign changes, and proactive planning instead of reactivity.

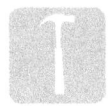 **For your toolkit... A positive leadership style is a cornerstone of success as well as a key retention strategy.**

Some of my additional management thoughts include:

- **Never forget what it's like to be in the trenches**. My first job was as a nurses' aide on evening shift in a skilled nursing home. I never want to forget the feelings I had having a charge nurse say "thank you" or getting angry at me for not be able to follow through on a task. I want to be sure I remember to manage others the way I would like to be managed.

- **Graciousness and common courtesy go a long way.** "Please," "thank you" and "I appreciate you working an extra shift." are not used nearly enough by healthcare managers. It takes two seconds to say please or thank you and the payback is endless. It also builds staff loyalty and willingness to help you achieve department goals.

- **Build trust.** Trust is a critical element to build with employees. It is also something that is earned, not given freely by employees and subordinates. When employees trust their manager, they will do anything to help accomplish goals and objectives.

- **Relationship management matters.** Most healthcare staff hate politics and consider management roles to be very "political". The reality is that management is all about managing relationships. You need to build strong allies in key departments to help you manage your work. Managing relationships builds trust as well as gives you an individual to network with to get the job done. Consider managing relationships to be the most important thing you do as a manager.

- **Being a good manager is not being popular.** Many decisions you make as a manager will be difficult and make at least some staff unhappy. You will need to learn to accept that making the right decision for your unit doesn't always make you popular with your staff.

- **Never ask someone to do something you wouldn't do yourself.** Employees need to know that you understand what it is like to be in the trenches. If you ask an employee to pick up trash, be sure you are willing to do it yourself before you ask. If you ask staff members to do only the things that you don't like to do, they will recognize it, and be resentful and unwilling to help. Staff will watch to see if you live up to what you ask of others.

- **If you ask staff members their opinions, be prepared to do something with the answers.** It is crucial to get staff feedback on issues related to care of patients and department goals and objectives. Keep in mind that if you ask opinions, the expectation is that you do something with the answers. Don't ask the question if you already know how you want to proceed—you will alienate employees. If you do ask for input, then provide follow-up to staff about how it was used in the final decision making process.

- **Manage by walking around.** This is a relatively old concept among business practices, but many healthcare managers don't use it. You can learn more about what is happening with your staff and what is working or not working on your unit in ten minutes than you can in a month of meetings. Get out of your office and talk to staff. You will be amazed at what you hear.

- **Delegate; then get out of the way.** Many healthcare managers believe in delegation, but can't actually let go of a process or project to let someone else take the reins. Meet with the staff to share the goal and outcome needed, provide the boundaries and any mandates that must be included. Give clear expectations and a completion date. Offer to be available for meetings and guidance. Then get out of the way and let the employees do their thing. Ask for feedback and follow-up. If they fail to deliver, you have learned a valuable lesson and so has the employee. More often than not, the staff member will deliver a completed project and you will have time to spend on other issues.

- **Embrace and manage change**. Transition is a steady, constant state, according to Mitchell Marks. Change never stops in healthcare; therefore, transition is always present. Learn to embrace it instead of fighting it. Learn about the change process and understand your feelings about each step. This will help you anticipate what may be your most difficult step of change when you encounter it. Embrace the change process with your staff as an opportunity to excel and achieve more that benefits patient care.

- **Be a risk taker**. Many healthcare managers are so worried about failure that they never take a chance on doing things differently. Failure is not a bad thing. Doing nothing means a missed opportunity. Learn to trust your intuition on how to proceed with new ideas, much as you have trusted it to tell you when a patient goes clinically bad. Some of the best things that have been implemented in healthcare happened because a manager took the risk to try something new.

- **Strive to become a leader, not just a manager**. Several business gurus like Deming and Drucker have identified the differences between management and leadership. One of the common threads in these business theories is that managers "do things right " but leaders "do the right things." Leaders are not always the most popular, but they are always respected.

- **Build bridges not kingdoms**. One of the most fatal mistakes you can make as a healthcare manager is to use your authority to build personal power and gain. Nothing will cause you to be disrespected more quickly than forgetting that being a manager is about being there for the staff members who work to support you-not just thinking of your own personal gains in a decision.

- **Being a good manager means empowerment.** As a manager you are not a problem solver as when you were as a staff worker. You need to get into the role of being a facilitator of thinking processes and a coach. Anyone can give advice, but it takes a good manager to empower employees to solve the problem on their own.

- **Communicate often and tell the truth:** You may not always be able to share good news, but ongoing honest and effective communication is critical to your success. Tell the truth. Never say never and remember to be human. If you lead with your heart first, then your head, you will do well as a manager.

- **Use the 24 hour rule:** Never make a difficult decision right away if you can avoid doing so. Taking an extra 24 hours to make a decision may save you lots of trouble (or embarrassment) later.

- **Remember that people are like popcorn:** People learn differently and at different speeds. People "pop" at different times. Some of your staff will understand exactly what you want them to do the first time you explain it. Others will take longer. Be patient with those who "pop" slower than others. It doesn't mean they're resisting –they just may not get it yet. Continue to make your request and explain the rationale. There are very few "duds" in employees. Eventually, most of them get it and are happy to help achieve department and organizational objectives.

- **Let go of vibrating poles:** There are multiple issues in healthcare organizations that can make you crazy. Our natural tendency is to try and control things so we can "fix" them. Most healthcare facilities are extremely dysfunctional, so we can't change anything. As we continue to try and control whatever is dysfunctional, the more frustrated we get, and still nothing changes. A healthcare organization is the equivalent of a vibrating pole. The temptation is to hang on to the pole to make it stop vibrating. In reality, that makes both you and the pole vibrate. The answer is to let go of the pole. Not easy to do in work settings, but the only thing that will save your sanity.

- **Make sure you fight over only silver bullets:** Because there are so many problems to solve in healthcare organizations, it is tempting to try and solve everyone of them. Choose "fighting issues" carefully. Every issue isn't worth going to the mat over. Pick the issues that will make the most difference to patient care, or that compromise your ethics or integrity. The rest probably don't matter that much. Ask yourself if this issue will make a difference in a year. If the answer is no, move on.

- **Remember that the patient is what matters the most:** It is easy to get lost in personnel, project and budget productivity issues. Try and remember that the reason you are a healthcare manager is to make a difference to the PATIENT. Always keep patients' needs as your central priority– you will rarely be faulted for doing so.

For your toolkit....Turner's Tips for Management Success

- *Never* forget what it's like to be in the trenches
- Graciousness and common courtesy go a long way
- Build trust
- Relationship management matters
- Being a good manager is not being popular
- Never ask someone to do something you wouldn't do yourself
- If you ask staff members their opinions, be prepared to do something with the answers
- Manage by walking around
- Delegate; then get out of the way
- Embrace and manage change
- Be a risk taker
- Strive to become a leader, not just a manager
- Build bridges not kingdoms
- Being a good manager means empowerment
- Communicate often and tell the truth
- Use the 24 hour rule
- Remember that people are like popcorn
- Let go of vibrating poles
- Make sure you fight over only silver bullets
- Remember that the patient is what matters the most

Turner Healthcare Associates, Inc. ©2005

Old Management vs. New management

Old way of managing (authoritarian)	New way of managing (participative)
Rigidly defined individual responsibilities	Flexible definition of responsibilities of team members via discussion and consensus
Fosters competition between individuals	Fosters cooperation and teamwork among members
Assumes that staff are passive, lack ambition and need controlling	Assumes that staff have motivation and readiness to direct behavior toward organizational goals
Management is to direct, control and motivate others	Arrange organizational conditions and operations so staff can achieve their on goals best by directing efforts toward organizational objectives
Quality is fine the way it is	Quality can and must improve
Checking data/reports ensures quality	Analysis and improving processes ensures quality
People cause defects and poor quality	Processes and systems cause defects and poor quality
Intuition and technology will solve problems	Collecting data and acting with knowledge will solve problems
Quality costs money	Quality saves money

Customers are problems	Customers are partners
Suppliers/vendors are problems	Suppliers/vendors are partners
We don't have time for quality and customer service	We don't have time not to have quality and customer service

Managing an Effective Team

The key to success as a supervisor or manager is the relationship between you and your work group. You are dependent on your group and you need it as much as it needs you. Organizations utilize the concept of synergy that teamwork can accomplish much more than its individual members can do by working alone. Most facilities cannot accomplish goals without teamwork, because the goals cannot e achieved by each supervisor or staff member individually.

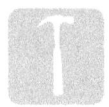 **For your toolkit.... The key to success as a supervisor or manager is the relationship between you and your work group.**

Calling a group a team doesn't make it a team. While teamwork is appropriate and desirable, a formal team structure is not always necessary. Creating a team for the sake of a team is a bad idea. Some healthcare tasks require teamwork and others require individual efforts. Teamwork is accomplished by making sure that cooperative behavior is positively reinforced.

In a team model of healthcare care, the collective team works towards the goal of managing the patient's care as directed by the physician. All care is coordinated by the case manager, and done in conjunction with the patient and involved family members. (Turner, 1998). The most effective healthcare work environment is one when people know when to work alone and when to ask for help. When you need to work with others to develop a solution to a complex problem, teams produce effective resolutions.

Bringing teams together increases the opportunities for receiving positive reinforcement between team members. Peers exert tremendous influence on the behavior of peers. If team members are taught how to positively reinforce one another for efforts made results achieved, the outcome will be effective teamwork. Team members have more contact with each other than do their managers, so reinforcement can be more frequent and since they are together while the work is occurring, reinforcement is likely to be immediate.

There are several essential elements that differentiate a team from a group of people. Within teams:

- The group members must have shared goals or a reason for working together
- The group members must be interdependent on each others' experience, abilities and commitment in order to achieve mutual goals
- The group members must be committed to the idea that working together leads to more effective decisions than working alone
- The group must be accountable as a functioning unit within a larger organizational context e.g. a hospital (Reilly,1974)

Making a group into a team means more than assuring the presence of these four elements for shared goals, interdependencies, commitment and accountability.

The aim of team building is to help a group evolve into a cohesive unit whose members not only share the same high expectations for accomplishing group tasks, but also trust and support one another and respect one another's individual differences. Teams that work together do well; teams with internal dissension don't work well together.

Nursing care teams are usually comprised of RNs, LVN/LPNs and CNAs. CNAs that work totally on their own to the exclusion of other team members will promote gaps in services and continuity of care. CNAs must work in collusion with other teams and departments to promote quality services. This also happens when licensed nurses working on their own exclude the CNAs. This results in the same disruption on quality of care. If you are not a nurse, you can still apply this concept to your team work. Quality care and efficient service means working together. If you are a supervisor, your task is to build a work group of willing, cooperative members who work together in a climate of acceptance support and trust. In short–a team.

Effective teams experience high productivity and morale. They tend to develop into their own social systems and experience high levels of group loyalty. Sometimes they develop "elitist" attitudes and see themselves as better than other groups. An effective team member has the following characteristics:

- Understands and is committed to team goals
- Is friendly, concerned and interested in others
- Acknowledges and confronts conflict openly
- Listens to others with understanding
- Includes others in the decision making process
- Recognizes and respects individual differences
- Contributes ideas and solutions
- Values and respects others' ideas and contributions
- Recognizes and rewards team efforts
- Encourages and appreciates feedback about team performance

Characteristics of effective team members

Effective team members:

- Support the team leader
- Help the team leader to succeed
- Ensure all viewpoints are explored
- Express opinions, both for and against an idea
- Compliment the team leader on team efforts
- Provide open honest and accurate information
- Understand personal and team roles

- Act in a positive and constructive manner
- Provide appropriate feedback
- Bring problems to the team
- Accept ownerships for team decisions
- Recognize that they each serve as team leaders at certain times
- Balance appropriate levels of participation
- Participate voluntarily
- Maintain confidentiality
- Show loyalty to the company, team leader and team
- View criticism as an opportunity to learn
- State problems, along with alternative solutions and options
- Give praise and recognition when warranted
- Operate within the parameters of team rules
- Confront the team leader when his/her behavior is not helping the team
- Share ideas freely and enthusiastically
- Encourage others to express their ideas fully
- Ask one another for opinions and listen to them
- Criticize ideas, not people
- Avoid disruptive behavior such as side conversations and inside jokes
- Avoid defensiveness when fellow team members disagree with their ideas
- Attend meetings regularly, promptly and enthusiastically

*Adapted from Supervisory Training Modules, Beverly Health

An effective team is one that can solve its own problems, and the ability to solve problems is predicated on an ability to identify and remove obstacles that deflect energy from those problems. When team members are expending energy on hidden agendas, internal conflicts, role ambiguity, confusion about the team's mission or value, than cannot focus their best efforts on solving the work-related problems that continually arise. The process of team building seeks to improve members' problem solving ability by enabling them to confront and manage the issues that hinder their functioning as a unit.

Team building does not happen quickly. It is an ongoing process and the personality of your team will change as employees grown in their jobs, add to the capabilities or gain or lose members. As a team leader you can help ensure the effectiveness of your team by helping your team members recognize their strengths and abilities. Team members need to be encouraged to develop their individual skills and give them the opportunity to stretch those skills. In addition, supervisors should focus on specific actions.

Treat your team members as well as you want them to treat patients. Make it clear that you expect them to treat each other with the same respect and level of service that they show their patients. Foster cooperation rather than competition between the members of your team. Be sure your team members know that no one stands alone. When they need support or a backup person, another team member should always be available.

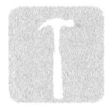 **For your toolkit... Treat your team members as well as you want them to treat patients.**

Be supportive and available to your team members. Let them know they can come to you any time with questions, problems, suggestions or ideas. Don't smother initiative and do get out of their way if they are doing a good job. Give suggestions, encouragement, support and a sympathetic ear when it is needed. Communication is the primary factor in developing teams. Teams are more than group with a single goal. They are composed of individuals with unique talents and personalities. It will take time to build the level of trust needed among the team member. It is communication that will make that a reality.

Understanding your group member dynamics will make you a more effective supervisor. Observing your members and getting to know them is the key to understanding their individual contributions to the group. Understanding the interactions among members will help you when you need to choose people for a new project. Taking advantage of member's natural skills and talents will help the team reach its goals.

Most people want the chance to be a member of a winning and productive team. They want the opportunity to contribute. That basic desire will help you to build a great team. It takes patience, but is worth the time and energy. The supervisor is an important part of the total team system. Highly effective work groups see their supervisors as:

- Supportive, friendly and helpful
- Having confidence in their ability and integrity
- Having high performance expectations
- Providing necessary training and coaching
- Viewing errors as learning opportunities rather than chances to criticize

Building a highly effective team starts with selecting and training qualified group members. The hiring process should include an interpersonal skills assessment of candidates to determine their abilities to work well with others in a team setting. Once they are hired, be sure they are thoroughly oriented to their job.

Then allow the team members the opportunity to influence group goals and the freedom to contribute to those goals. This will allow you to concentrate on solving problems that interfere with goal achievement and building a positive identify for the work team. This identity must end up as a "collective ego" of individuals. Self-interested individuals destroy teamwork success. Each team member must be professional, know their role and perform at their highest level. Supervisors must train each team member in such as way as to allow each team member to provide necessary skills. The trust and loyalty of the group will develop over time as they work together.

Supervisors must create team building in four areas. Providing support is crucial. These are things you do to increase or maintain each group member's sense of personal worth and importance as a team member such as providing encouragement and recognition for good performance, speaking out on behalf of group members and referring others directly to group members to answer questions or solve problems.

Promoting interaction between members encourages relating. These are things you do create or maintain a network of interpersonal relationships among group members, such as sponsoring or encouraging group social events, holding work group meetings and arranging lunch breaks so group members can be together.

Emphasizing group goals are the things you do to create a high level of awareness and commitment to deliver a product or service to your customers by creating, changing, clarifying and gaining acceptance of group goals. This is typically done best through the involvement and participation of group members.

The last area supervisors must focus on is facilitating group task accomplishment. These are things you do to provide effective work methods, facilities, equipment and schedules for accomplishing group goals. This will include solving problems that your group experiences with other groups it interfaces with to achieve goals. Sometimes this involves conflict resolution between team members.

These four areas of involvement are essential for an effective team. However, the supervisor is not the only person that needs to contribute to the group in these areas. Team members help each other in highly effective groups. The supervisor's attitude and involvement patterns tend to be mirrored in the behavior of the group members. Therefore the responsibility for group success and effectiveness is shifted to all members of the team. Supervisors need to manage team members more as a coach than a boss. This means that staff needs to understand in behavioral terms what they are do to. You must clarify what group members are to do in a coaching way:

Supervisory behaviors	Coaching behaviors
Hand out assignments	Develop a positive reinforcement plan
Tell people how to do a job	Give performance feedback
Keep people on task	Share information

Find and punish poor performance	Mediate reinforcement between team members
Protect organization information	Deliver positive reinforcement for decision making, creative solutions, cooperation and initiative.

Changing behavior requires many reinforcements of the new behavior before new habits are successfully entrenched. You can not reinforce a team. You can only reinforce team member behaviors.

You can reward a team, but it works best when all members are contributing equally. It is the supervisor's responsibility to apply consequences to team members in such a way that everybody is reinforced appropriately for their contributions to the team. It is critical that the criteria for receiving reinforcement and rewards are clear and achievable. If they are not, skepticism, cynicism and bitterness among team members may occur. The best way to empower team members is gradually and systematically.

You can encourage team development by providing support, promoting interaction, emphasizing goals, and facilitating task accomplishment. Be willing to share goal setting decision making, problem solving and control with your group. Once you have an effective team, everyone's job will be easier, and more enjoyable–especially yours.

Most people want the chance to be a member of a winning team. They want to contribute to the group. You, as the supervisor, must facilitate and reinforce teamwork and provide your staff with the tasks and projects to challenge them successfully. You will also reap the benefits and satisfaction of team building and discover the value of teams.

Characteristics of Effective Team Leaders

Effective team leaders:

- Communicate
- Are open, honest and fair
- Make decisions with input from others
- Acts consistently
- Give the team members the information they need to do their jobs
- Set goals and emphasize them
- Keep focused through follow-up
- Listen to feedback and ask questions
- Show loyalty to the company and to the team members
- Create an atmosphere for growth
- Have wide visibility
- Give praise and recognition
- Criticize constructively and address problems
- Develop plans
- Share their mission and goals
- Display tolerance and flexibility
- Demonstrate assertiveness
- Exhibit willingness to change
- Treat team members with respect
- Make themselves available and accessible
- Want to take charge
- Accept ownership for team decisions
- Set guidelines for how team members are to treat one another
- Represent the team and fight "the good fight" when appropriate

*Adapted from Supervisory Training Modules, Beverly Health

Teamwork is demanding off the individual members. Supervisors and team leaders need to be cognizant of this fact and appreciate the effort required of group members.

Characteristics of an Effective Team:

- Team members share a sense of purpose or common goals, and each team member is willing to work toward achieving these goals.
- The team is aware of an interested in its own processes and examining norms operating within the team.
- The team identifies its own resources and uses them, depending on its needs. The team willingly accepts the influence and leadership of the members whose resources are relevant to the immediate task.
- The team members continually try to listen to and clarify what is being said and show interest in what others say and feel.
- Differences of opinion are encouraged and freely expressed. The team does not demand narrow conformity or adherence to formats that inhibit freedom of movement and expression.
- The team is willing to surface conflict and focus on it until it is resolved or managed in a way that does not reduce the effectiveness of those involved.
- The team exerts energy toward problem solving rather than allowing it to be drained by interpersonal issues or competitive struggles.
- Roles are balanced and shared to facilitate both the accomplishment of tasks and feelings of team cohesion and morale.
- To encourage risk taking and creativity, mistakes are treated as sources of learning rather than reasons for punishment.
- The team is responsive to the changing needs of its members and to the external environment to which it is related.
- Team members are committed to periodically evaluating the team's performance.
- The team is attractive to its members who identify with it and consider it a source of both professional and personal growth.
- Developing a climate of trust is recognized as the crucial element for facilitating all of the above elements.

*Adapted from Beverly Health Supervisory Training Modules, 2005

Each team member and discipline must function within their scope of practice. Every state has a specific scope of practice for licensed healthcare staff.

These scopes are regulatory in nature and identify what the practitioner can and cannot do within their specific role. It is both illegal and unsafe to ask a team member to do something outside of their specific scope of practice. It is incumbent on every practitioner to be familiar with their professional scope of practice. Saying you didn't know about your scope of practice requirements will do nothing to protect you in a malpractice lawsuit. State scope of practice regulations are legal requirements of how you can practice your healthcare specialty and/or what staff are allowed to do (or forbidden from doing).

Each person on the team has certain responsibilities to fulfill when working. Those responsibilities usually are determined by the charge personnel on each shift. Because each shift of staff has different responsibilities depending on the time of day and the type of unit, these responsibilities vary between shifts.

Each team member is responsible for tasks according to their individual scope of practice. The team leader is charged with making appropriate decisions that result in effective use of the team. A successful team has all members working together and communicating well with each other. Tasks are completed, not forgotten, and changing patient conditions are promptly reported and managed.

Routine members of the patient care team include:

- Dietary
- Infection control
- Nurse
- Pharmacist
- Physician
- Clinical case manager
- Radiology technologist
- Clinical Laboratory Scientist
- Discharge planner

Standards of practice and role-based competencies drive different roles, functions and tasks. Standards of practice and competent performance are defined by several organizations, including hospitals as well as regulatory and specialty agencies. Standard practices and skill-based competencies are defined by hospital policy and directed toward the ongoing commitment to quality improvement and patient satisfaction.

Standards for performance are also defined by individual job descriptions for each team member. Facility job descriptions list specific tasks and functions for each role. Performance evaluations are geared to specific job description requirements, tasks and functions for each role. Standards of practice are also defined by state and federal mandates and are regulatory in nature. You can review the standards of competent performance for your type of licensure and specialty on your state board web site.

Accountability is also a function of team work. Each team member is held accountable and must be responsible to carrying out the physician orders within their scope of practice. Members of a team have accountability not only to the patient, but also the patient's family, the physician, the organization, the payer and other team members.

Commitment is part of being a team. Each team member must be committed to the goals of the team and the organization. Each team member is accountable for and committed to implementing the patient's plan of care within each discipline and scope of practice. They must utilize their skills to the overall benefit of the patient. A commitment also exists between each team member, the patient and the patient's family, as well as to providing a high quality of care. All members must be committed to positive patient outcomes as well as cost-effective patient care.

Newly constructed teams go through several stages before they work well together. Several decades ago, Tuckman created a model for team functioning that is well known in management circles. (2012) Tuckman lists four stages of team development. Each team goes through these stages, some more quickly than others. Ultimately, most teams are effective, but need to learn how to work together. These stages are:

- Forming: getting started; getting to know each other, not sure what to do
- Storming: going in circles, having trouble working together; focused on end goal instead of process of getting work done.
- Norming: getting on course, now know each other; identify goal and work together

- Performing: work at full speed ahead; working together to achieve goal; use feedback to make changes and look for ways to improve

Even if you are a healthcare manager and part of an administrative team, your team members still go through these four stages. Some teams are dysfunctional and never get out of the storming phase. Committees and unit teams that are effectively have successfully worked through all four stages and remain in the performing stage for the long term. Whenever a new team member joins the group, it is common for the team to go back through storming and norming stages again before getting back to performing.

As with everything else related to healthcare, communication is critical between team members. Staff and team members will tend to perform functions that support the mission of the organization and unit if they:

- Have clearly defined goals
- Recognize how they treat each other will affect how they relate to patients
- Recognize the team leader and his/her functions and responsibilities
- Agree on the purpose and functions of the team
- Are clear on who is responsible, who has authority and who is accountable for what tasks and functions
- Have open and honest communication
- Conflict is dealt with honestly and openly
- Welcome and accept new members
- Value all team members
- Understand all team member roles and tasks and define them for the entire team
- Provide continual information within and for the team

Teams work best if team leaders are:

- Supportive of team members' sense of self-worth and importance of each members role
- Open to ideas and suggestions of how to accomplish team workload

- Embracing high standards of performance that are clearly communicated
- Encouraging all members to express ideas and to be valued by other members
- Ensuring that team members have what they need to perform their role and tasks-equipment, knowledge, resources, skills
- Coaching team members at their particular level of ability to enhance performance (one size coaching DOES NOT fit all)
- Placing emphasis on problem solving, not blaming
- Recognizing obstacles and change are facts of life for teams

It is important for team leaders and members to know when to:
- Empower all team members
- Educate when conditions are new or changed
- Coach before, during and after a first experience
- Counsel when problems damage performance
- Confront problems are persistent or the person is failing
- Give feedback early and give it often

Teams require effective personal communication:
- Goal is to create understanding
- Listening is more important than talking
- Nonverbal communication is 98% of process
- Two way communication is preferred
- One way communication may be necessary if there is a crisis

Delegation to other team members:
- Team leader identifies tasks to be delegated
- Team member's responsibility is to complete tasks AND report back to team leader
- Must be within licensed specialty practice scope
- Is not "dumping" unsavory tasks
- Must be sure team member is competent and has equipment/supplies to do task

- Is an opportunity to teach team members new skills by demonstrating procedure or tasks?

 **For your toolkit... When working with a team, listening is more important than talking**

Effective Delegation

All supervisors and managers wonder at some point why they have so much work to complete and no one to assist with it. Reasons for this perception include:

- Not enough time
- I'd rather do it myself
- I can't trust a subordinate will do it correctly
- I can't give my work to someone else, because my boss will think I can't do it
- It's my job
- My subordinates already have too much to do

No matter how effective you are as a supervisor, there is a limit to the capacity you can accomplish as a working supervisor. Successful supervisors know when and what to delegate. Delegation is the assignment of authority for the completion of tasks to others. This allows completion and achievement of organizational goals. Effective supervisors learn the art of effective delegation and in doing so has resulted in "win-win" for both the supervisor and the subordinate.

One of the major concepts of delegation is to provide your subordinates with the necessary information and authority to complete the tasks assigned, but you retain the responsibility for the final achievement of the goals or outcome. In doing this, you and your subordinates gain these benefits:

- Increased span of responsibility
- Increased time to spend on planning
- Staff development of subordinates
- Increased motivation
- Increased productivity and efficiency

You "win" as a supervisor in that as you increase the responsibilities of your subordinates, you expand your own ability to manage more effectively through increased planning and decision making. Your subordinates "win" through the application of skills they have learned and the empowerment gained in solving work problems. Both of you "win" when your value to the organization increases and the job satisfaction of the team is enhanced.

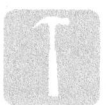
For your toolkit… As you increase the responsibilities of your subordinates, you expand your own ability to manage more effectively

Now that you understand the idea and value of delegation, how do you go about doing it? Many supervisors believe that delegating means assigning parts of their work to someone else that they don't want to do. This is not delegating. It is dumping. To properly delegate to others you must first analyze what tasks you can safely, legally and appropriately delegate. Consider training, certification or licensure requirements when evaluating this. Determine the authority needed for the job and how much can be delegated. Consider such things as requesting information from others in the organization. Can your subordinate have access to the same information? Can s/he represent you?

You must then determine who the "right person for the job" is. Consider the following components. Does the work belong to a particular position? Does the task delegated fit well with duties already performed, and thus would logically fit there? Who has the interest and/or ability? Who has the time? Is there a part-time person who could take on a new task and/or project? Is there a person whose workload has periods that are cyclic or lighter? Determine the controls to ensure the task is completed successfully. How much control will be needed to ensure completion of the task delegated? Consider such things as establishment off deadlines and check-in dates.

There are certain tasks you cannot delegate to others as a supervisor. These include things like discipline or subordinates or implementations of policies. Other examples are duties which require licensure or other specific credentialing or access to data e.g. payroll. You may not be able to delegate certain tasks to others because they have not been trained, such as completing a specific form or process. Tailor your delegation to fit your subordinates' abilities while yet allowing them the freedom to expand their skills.

You must also assess how much authority you can delegate to others based on the tasks assigned. For example, if you ask someone to investigate a work related injury and make recommendations to prevent further incidents, then you must also ensure they have the authority to conduct the investigation on your behalf. The nature and amount of authority should be clearly defined and communicated to the subordinate. Delegating a portion of your authority to a subordinate does not relieve you of your responsibility to your boss and the organization to ensure these duties are properly completed.

In addition to determining what tasks you can delegate and how much authority is needed to complete them, you must also establish controls for the type of work assigned. The methods you choose for control should be suited to the nature of the assignment and to the person to whom you have given the assignment. In some cases, periodic written reports may be required. In other cases, spot checks or verbal briefings may be enough. Once you have determined the controls needed to complete the tasks assigned, clearly communicate those to the subordinate.

Delegation has several steps to ensure delegation with effective results.

Explain why the job is important. Explain the end results needed and let the staff member determine who the task will be completed her/himself. Delegate in terms of results and outcomes, not process or methods. Clearly define the staff members' authority and parameters that they have when completing the task. Agree on a deadline and time frame with the staff member. Ask for feedback to ensure the staff member understands the task completely. Provide for controls to ensure the staff member is on the right track. Follow-up and check on progress yourself. Give support and leave an opportunity for the staff member to come back to you if they have questions.

Once an assignment is completed, be sure to give your subordinate credit for a job well done. You take responsibility if the assignment was less than successful. Let your subordinate know how well they did. If needed, review the original directions and discuss how to accomplish the assignment more effectively in the future. If the assignment was not completed accurately, find out what went wrong and why. Ask for your subordinates feedback with regard to the assignment and if they will do another in the future.

These skills discussed will prepare you to be a more effective delegator. To prepare for your next opportunity to delegate, try imagining yourself preparing to delegate to a specific subordinate. Picture the person, now think about the right approach to use in conveying this assignment to this person. Imagine how the person will respond. How will you go about getting feedback from this person about the assignment? How will you communicate their authority? What check dates and processes or deadlines will you establish? How will you ensure understanding of the assignment?

Delegation Dos and Don'ts

DO	DON'T
Encourage free flow of information to subordinates	Hoard information
Focus on results	Emphasize methods
Delegate through dialogue	Do al the talking yourself
Fix firm deadlines	Leave timeframes unclear or uncertain
Make sure the person has all the necessary resources	Half delegate by giving assignments without the needed tools and information
Delegate the entire task to one person	Delegate half the task
Give advice without interfering	Fail to point out pitfalls
Build controls into the process of delegating	Impose controls as an afterthought
Back up those delegated to in legitimate disputes	Leave persons to fight their own battles on your behalf
Give the delegate full credit for his/her accomplishments	Hog the glory or look for a scapegoat

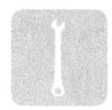 **Turner Delegation Self Assessment Checklist©**

Check all that apply:

1. Your workload has prevented you from taking regular vacations.
2. You feel overworked frequently.
3. You leave jobs unfinished.
4. You take work home most nights and weekends.
5. It always seems you have more work than your subordinates.
6. Planning is a low priority task for you.
7. You have no time for outside activities.
8. In the past week, you have engaged in detail work that isn't your job.
9. You do your subordinates' work for them frequently.
10. Crises and problems are more common in your job than opportunities.
11. Often you haven't had time to fully explain a task to your subordinate.
12. You frequently have problems meeting your boss's deadlines.
13. You like to keep your hands in your old job.
14. You are a perfectionist– and proud of it!
15. You wish you had more time in your personal life.
16. You can't think of your top three current work goals.
17. You believe in giving subordinates only the information they need to do their specific jobs.
18. You rarely elicit the opinions of your subordinates about anything.
19. In your opinion, your subordinates are not to be trusted with too much information.
20. It is hard for you to accept ideas offered by someone else.
21. You get the feeling that sometimes your subordinates are trying to undermine you.

22. You believe your subordinates are coasting.

23. Your subordinates' think how something is done is more important than what is achieved.

24. Your staff refuses to make any decisions without consulting you first.

25. Your staff comes to you for advice on their work more than necessary.

26. Your staff exceeds their authority regularly.

27. Your staff acts according to the literal rather than the spirit of an assignment.

28. Sometimes, your staff consults with you after the fact about significant actions.

29. None of your staff could fill in for you if you got run over by a bus.

30. Your staff turns work assignments back to you and you accept them.

31. Your staff wouldn't work at all if you weren't there to push them to do tasks.

32. Your staff has skills essentially unchanged from a year ago.

33. Staff rarely comes to you with new ideas or new ways of doing their jobs.

Turner Healthcare Associates, Inc, © 1999

Evaluating and Critiquing Performance

Most people think of performance evaluations as something that happens once a year or if you make a mistake. In reality, evaluating performance is a process that happens over time. While supervisors and managers do formal performance evaluations, charge personnel and team leaders routinely evaluate performance of their team members. A performance evaluation is an opportunity to assess the demonstrated performance of team members and staff over a period of time. The evaluation communicates the assessment and expectations for the future. The document is a way to review the past and look toward the future using the performance evaluation process.

Numerous studies have been done in different industries about what is most important to people about working. Probably one of the most well known books on the subject is *Art of Managing People* by Philip L. Hunsacker and Anthony L. Allesandria. The two most frequently mentioned responses to all these studies were communication and recognition. People have a desire for accurate, timely information. People want to be "let in on things" or "in the loop" for real time information. Not providing information makes staff members think you are deliberately keeping bad news from them. The second desire is to be recognized for a job well done. A "pat on the back" is a way of formally recognizing the employee and makes them aware that their supervisor knows they did a good job. Staff expects communication and recognition from their direct supervisor. Even if you are not a designated supervisor, but function in the role of team leader or charge personnel, staff will expect informal feedback about their performance.

The reasons that actual performance evaluation is such a significant process are because it addresses these two important employee needs for communication and recognition. It gives a supervisor the chance to accurately communicate how a staff member is performing their job. It is also a time for both the staff member and the supervisor to restate expectations and set new goals. Performance evaluations give the supervisor an opportunity to recognize staff performance and praise strengths as well as identify areas to improve. This should be happening on an ongoing basis so that getting a performance evaluation should have no surprises for the staff member.

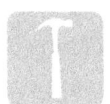 **For your toolkit... Getting a performance evaluation should mean no surprises for the staff member.**

Communication is a large part of the performance evaluation process. As discussed in the section on effective communication, words are important but how we communicate beyond just word selection makes up the bulk of our communication. To be accurate in communication in the performance evaluation process means that the supervisor or team leader must accurately assess the staff members' performance. This means concentrating on job performance–not the staff member's personality–when making this assessment.

Timely

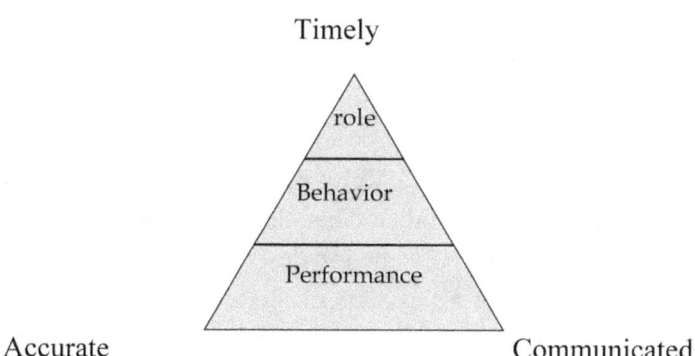

Accurate   Communicated

Performance evaluations can be thought of as a triangle. It must be accurate, communicated and timely. Most employees know when their performance evaluations are due because it is important to them. Completing them in a timely fashion builds credibility for the supervisor and respect of the employees. When communicating to staff, be sure that communication is not just one sided. It is an exchange between you and your associates. In this process the supervisor should solicit input, comments and suggestions from the employee.

When completing a performance evaluation, start the process early. Be on time with completion of the evaluation. Review the employee's file for commendations, discipline, and memos for follow up. Do this so you can consider the total performance. Remember that it is ultimately a positive thing if a staff member overcomes a previous performance problem. Review the employee's job description to assure it is still accurate and to assist you in considering the entire job and all its various responsibilities. Assess job performance objectively, not the staff member's personality or attitude. Assess how the employee has performed the job, not just whether you think they are a "nice person."

Your objectivity is enhanced when there are job duties that can be counted or measured, e.g. attendance, number of students preceptored, etc. Consider the staff members performance for the entire time period. Do not base your assessment on only the most recent weeks or months. You are assessing performance for the entire year. Use specific examples to describe positive and negative performance. Use examples to clarify ad support your position and promote credibility.

Schedule time to meet with the employee. This demonstrates your respect for the process and the staff member. This also gives the staff member time to prepare for the meeting. Review the job description in advance of meeting with the employee. Consider all aspects of the job duties. Meet in a private and comfortable place behind closed doors. This eliminates interruptions and maintains privacy. Explain the purpose of the discussion and set the stage for an open, honest, cordial discussion. Praise the employee's strengths and identify areas to improve. Balance the discussion with comments on both areas.

Encourage the staff member to participate with input and comments. The contact should not be a one-sided monologue. The discussion requires input from the staff member as well as the supervisors. Give the employee every opportunity to participate in the process by listening and not interrupting. Focus your comments on the employee's performance, not personality. There should be no surprises for the employee during this discussion. Recognition and corrective action should take place as soon as needed-not save for the performance evaluation meeting.

Avoid confrontation and argument with the employee. Listen with objectivity and stress performance, not personality or attitude. Assess the employees past demonstrated performance, but emphasize the future and professional growth. Restate your expectations. Don't "save" communicating expectations for these meetings, but rather use the time to reinforce those you have already shared with the employee. Set new goals, considering progress, growth, future, and employee development. Establish a plan and time table to meet those objectives with the employee. Be specific and monitor that the time table is being met by the employee. Be sure the employee is aware of the effects of not satisfying performance standards. Employees deserve to know the consequences of not performing to expectations. Remember to say "thank you" for your associate's participation in the meeting and their contribution for the year.

There are specific ways to describe both positive and negative employee behaviors in a written performance evaluation. Be sure to always support the adjectives used with specific examples of the staff member's behavior. Below are listed some words and phrases that can be used for specifically describing both positive and negative behaviors.

Positive Behaviors	Negative Behaviors
Methodical	Needs many explanations
Generates enthusiasm	Perfectionist
Willing to accept difficult assignments	Slow to get things done; resists difficult materials
Pays attention to deadlines	Overreacts to criticism
Avoids risks	Tends to day dream
Gets tasks done	Unprepared
Accountable for own work	Shifts blame to others
Sets and completes goals	Disorganized
Sensitive when showing disapproval	Unfriendly to patients; inefficient
Willing to help others succeed	Does not check work before submission

Obtains needed information	Resists changes
Shares information with others	Disrupts meetings
Maintains high standards	Takes shortcuts
Flexible	Sensitive to criticism
Becomes adaptable to those in authority	Resist participation in team; displays superior attitude
Gives recognition to others	Overuses enthusiasm
Takes on challenges	Displays frustration
Works calmly in unpredictable environment	Under pressure becomes soft and persuadable
Good organizer	Easily intimidated
Good listener; team player	Fails to communicate information, directions, feelings
Innovative	Shows little imagination
Makes good decisions quickly	Makes decisions too fast
Diplomatic with people	Abrupt with others

Providing Discipline to staff members

Formal progressive discipline is a last resort for sharing expectations with employees. If employee performance is a problem, then numerous discussions and clarification of performance expectations should take place before the disciplinary process begins. Just the word "discipline" strikes fear in even the most confident managers. It doesn't need to. While you probably will never look forward to taking disciplinary action, you can get to a point where you are comfortable and confident in what you are doing.

Progressive discipline is used to correct a deficiency in conduct, performance, or a violation of policy in an effort to meet established standards of job performance to preserve employment, and to encourage staff to behave sensibly and safely at work. Progressive discipline is actually a continually forward focused instruction and education process. In using discipline as a form of training, it would be appropriate to reward staff that observes facility rules that meet or exceed performance standards with praise and advancement. It is also then appropriate to discipline those staff members who do not measure up to facility rules and performance standards so they can be educated as to what acceptable performance and behavior is. Staff needs to hear what they are doing right as well as feedback on problematic personnel issues.

Chaos would ensue if there were no rules in the workplace. Most staff sees discipline as a way to preserve order and safety in the work place. It is reasonable and expected that an organization has staff working towards common organizational goals and standards. Staff expects just and equal treatment in which the discipline is in line with the performance problem or misconduct. The action must fit the infraction, and all staff members who are disciplined for an action must be treated equitably and fairly. Staff expects reasonable policies and consistent application of those policies.

Most staff members are conscientious, dependable and want to do a good job. They infrequently or never are subject to disciplinary action. When these individuals have a performance problem, it is generally an isolated incident which is quickly corrected with counseling or disciplinary action. There is a small percentage of staff that does cause disciplinary problems. Ongoing performance and conduct problems can result from lack of interest, lack of effort, problems getting along with others or problems at home. Part of a supervisor's job is to help staff adjust to their work. If the supervisor is a good leader, shows a sincere interest in staff and makes work enjoyable, the staff is far less likely to break rules or cause problems. Each facility has specific progressive discipline policies. If you are a supervisor and expected to administer progressive discipline, become familiar with the policy *before* you need to implement it. The stress and urgency of an actual disciplinary situation is not when you want to be reading the policy for the first time.

Most facilities have a policy that starts with a clarification of performance expectations. If problems continue, the employee received a verbal warning. Facilities use either one or two written warnings, and then an employee is terminated. There are instances where termination is immediate for gross misconduct such as threatening another employee, being under the influence of a chemical substance or lying during your interview or on your employment application.

One of the most important aspects of the disciplinary process is to determine whether it is truly called for. A complete and impartial investigation into the situation must be conducted before discipline is issued. Usually, the more information is at your disposal, the clearer the decision generally is. Once your investigation has revealed that the employee has committed a known policy violation, it is time to ascertain what action to take. Employees are often placed on suspension until the investigation is completed. The usual timeframe for this type of suspension is up to three regularly scheduled days, but varies by facility.

Verbal warnings are not mandatory, but are usually issued prior to a written warning, particularly if the infraction is minor in nature. Ironically, verbal warnings are actually documented in writing for the employee file. Written warnings are usually issued once the employee has received a verbal warning already and failed to correct the deficiency, has committed a more serious infraction which warrants more than a verbal warning or has one or more prior verbal or written warnings. Termination happens infrequently and is used when no other alternative exists to deal with the infraction. Termination is rarely immediate, and is usually contemplated after the investigation is completed.

If you must conduct a disciplinary meeting with an employee, schedule it after the investigation is completed. Make an appointment, and ensure complete privacy. Complete the necessary paperwork prior to the meeting and have it ready, including paychecks and forms if it is a termination. Review the paperwork with the employee, and explain why the action is being taken. Get the necessary signatures and provide the employee with a copy of the disciplinary action document. If the employee has been terminated, have them discreetly escorted out of the facility. After the meeting has taken place, document the conversation, and submit all paperwork for additional signatures and processing.

Progressive discipline is not much fun for anyone involved in it. It is much easier to coach and supervise employees instead of disciplining them. Remember that proper training, education and supervisory support will go a long way in preventing the need for disciplinary action. Discipline should be used only as necessary and then as a corrective action. It is much easier to stop a small problem and avoid much larger issues.

Decision making

Part of being a successful manager or supervisor is to have the competencies needed to achieve goals. Katz identified three essential management skill sets: technical, human and conceptual. (Robbins) Technical skills are those that encompass the ability to apply specialized knowledge or expertise. Extensive formal education is needed to learn the special knowledge and practices. Human skills are those that demonstrate ability to work with, understand and motivate other people, both individually and in groups. Many managers are technically proficient but interpersonally incompetent. Since managers get things done through other people, they must have good human skills to communicate, motivate and delegate. Managers that are poor listeners unable to understand the needs of others or have difficulty managing conflicts will not be effective as managers.

A key concept that affects managers' abilities to get things done is their ability to manage problem solving and make decisions. Problem solving and decision making are based on perception. People don't *see* reality. They *interpret* what they see and call it reality. Perception is defined as the process by which individuals organize and interpret their sensory impressions in order to give meaning to their environment. However, what one perceives can be substantially different from objective reality. (Robbins)

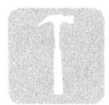 **For your toolkit.... People don't *see* reality. They *interpret* what they see and call it reality.**

There are numerous factors that influence perception. Attitudes, motives, interests, experience and expectations all affect how people view a situation. In a given situation, issues like time, and setting (personal or workplace) when influencing perception. The target that is being observed also has factors that affect individuals' perceptions. Novelty, motion, sounds, size, background and proximity all influence individual perceptions about a given experience. These factors become significant when managers are evaluating workplace situations and making decisions. (Robbins)

There is a link between perception and decision making. Managers and individuals in an organization make decisions from choices among two or more alternatives. Decision making occurs as a reaction to a problem. A discrepancy exists between a current state of affairs and a desired state, requiring consideration of alternative courses of action. (Robbins) Unfortunately, most problems don't come neatly packaged with a label on them. One person's problem is another person's satisfactory state of affairs. Every decision requires interpretation and evaluation of information. Data must be screened, processed and interpreted to allow evaluation.

Because people perceive experiences differently, no two people approach decision making the same way. However, there is an optimum way of making decisions. The Optimizing Decision Making Model describes how individuals should behave in order to maximize an outcome. (Robbins) There are six steps to this process. The first step requires recognition that a decision needs to be made. The existence of a problem brings about this recognition. The second step is to identify the decision criteria. Once an individual has determined the need for a decision, the criteria that will be important in making the decision must be identified. In healthcare, important criteria are often considered to be length of stay, productivity, overtime, staffing matrices, and patient outcomes. The criteria represent what the decision maker thinks is relevant to the decision. In this step, the only criteria evaluated are those the decision maker considers relevant. Therefore, different people will have different decision criteria.

The next step is to allocate weights to the criteria. Not all criteria are equally important. It is necessary to weight the factors in order to prioritize their importance in the decision. All the criteria are relevant, but some are more relevant than others. The decision maker can weight criteria numerically or with other measures. The result is to allow decision makers to use their personal preferences to prioritize the relevant criteria and to indicate the criteria's relative degree of importance by assigning a weight to each.

The fourth step is to develop alternatives. The decision maker lists all the viable alternatives that could possibly succeed in resolving the problem. Not attempt is made to appraise alternatives, but rather only to list them. Step five involves evaluating the alternatives. Once the alternatives have been identified, the decision maker must critically evaluate each one. The strengths and weaknesses of each alternative will become evident when compared against the criteria and weights established in the previous steps. Evaluation of each alternative is done by appraising it against the weighted criteria.

The last step is to select the best alternative. Technically, this should be easy. The decision maker simply chooses the alternative that generated the largest total score. However, good decisions in the healthcare industry are rarely so clearly identified. For most people, the optimizing model is usually the exception, not the rule. Few important decisions are simple or unambiguous. Some managers look for solutions that suffice rather than optimize, which injects biases and prejudices into the decision process. Others rely on intuition. Most managers and supervisors attempt to make rational decisions.

Rationality refers to choices that are consistent and value maximizing. Rational decision making implies that the decision maker can be fully objective and logical with a clear goal.(Robbins) Rationality and the optimizing model assume there is no conflict over goals and that all options are known and identified, with constant and unchanging criteria and preferences. Rational decision makers would choose the alternative that gives the maximum benefits or maximizes the decision outcome. Decision making is not just an analysis of facts. There is an element of "gut feel" to the process, especially when it comes to knowing when you have reached the point where you have sufficient facts on which to base a decision with a minimum of risk. This "gut feel" often separates the effective from the ineffective manager. (Robbins)

Steps in Optimizing Decision Making

1. Ascertain the need for a decision
2. Identify the decision criteria
3. Allocate weights to the criteria
4. Develop alternatives
5. Evaluate alternatives
6. Select the best alternative

Problem Solving

Problem solving requires good decision making. The end result of decision making by individuals and groups is driven by their ability to solve problems. Although we would like to think otherwise, problems exist for all groups that work together. Problem solving is a process. Robbins identifies a nine step process of problem solving (2012)

The first step is to identify the apparent problem versus the root problem. The apparent problem is what you think caused the issue. The root problem is what actually went wrong. The root problem is rarely the apparent problem. It is important to uncover the root problem, because it may be much more significant that the apparent problem. This is called the "iceberg effect." (Robbins) Many problem solving teams have been established to identify the actual root cause of a problem. Identifying the root cause of a problem allows all factors to be evaluated and corrected and minimizes blame of specific individuals.

 **For your toolkit... The apparent problem is what you think caused the issue. The root problem is what actually went wrong.**

The second step is to identify key players needed in the resolution of the problems. Problem solving teams try to bring all involved or affected parties together. The group then can define a problem statement. Often this statement is not the same as the original apparent problem. The fourth step is to collect information and data about the situation. It is important to collect and analyze data with the idea of resolving the issue. There are organizations that continually collect data, but rarely do anything with the information. This is known as "analysis paralysis" and does not move toward problem solving and resolution.

The fifth step is to share the data with ALL the stakeholders. This means sharing the data (not *just* the interpretation of the data) with *everyone* potentially affected by the problem and the resolution. This is usually a lot of people. Those who schedule meetings tend to limit the number of participants and focus only on having managers attend. Unfortunately, it is the front line staff that usually has first hand experience with the problem and can help with potential solutions. Be sure to include everyone who can help resolve a problem.

Once the larger group is gathered, explain both the apparent problem and the root cause, if known. Have all participants brainstorm solutions. During brainstorming, include all suggestions no matter how outlandish. Brainstorming is the time for listing all ideas without judgment or commentary. The group can evaluate them later.

Using the elimination technique, isolate the best ideas and create a plan of action.

Inform ALL stakeholders of this plan and ask for feedback *before* implementing it. Make revisions to the plan and then determine an implementation strategy that works for ALL the stakeholders. Faulty implementation of a plan can make a good decision ineffective.

Effective implementation of a plan can make a debatable choice successful. Solving the root problem is only half of the solution. Implementation of a plan is what will complete the cycle.

When teams work together on problem solving, they often get stuck in terms of their ability to move through a problem to the solution.

You can identify the team behaving as "stuck" by symptoms such as:
- Lack of progress
- Canceling meetings
- Angry exchanges between members
- Loss of energy
- Helplessness/victimization
- Lack of purpose/identity
- Dishonesty and lack of candor
- Cynicism and mistrust
- Personal attacks made behind team members' backs
- Finger pointing

Getting the team unstuck involves revisiting the purpose of team, identifying small "wins' and progress steps. Sometimes you can also search out new information and approaches. In rare situations, you may need to consider changing team members, including the team leader.

Many times the "stuckness" is caused by conflict. This is usually because team members have different ideas of what the team goal is or how to get there. Because tasks toward problem resolution affect more than one person/group, what works successfully in one spot of the organization is a disaster in another. There are often scarce resources, which cause team members to get frustrated if their unit does not obtain some of those scarce resources. Hospital organizational structure may also impede solutions and problem solving due to dysfunctional senior management teams or bureaucratic delays. All of these issues can cause conflict for teams.

Symptoms of a "Stuck" Team

- Loss of energy
- Helplessness/victimization
- Lack of purpose/identity
- Dishonesty and lack of candor
- Cynicism and mistrust
- Personal attacks made behind team members' backs
- Finger pointing

When managing the conflict in a team, remember that problem solving efforts must include members from conflicting groups. This does not mean that groups should point fingers at each other, but rather calmly discuss their perceptions and differences. It is also helpful to rotate team members among different teams to facilitate understanding. The best example I have experienced with this in my career is to have an RN that has worked in the intensive care unit (ICU) transfer down to the Emergency Department (ED) as a float or per diem staff member. Once an ICU nurse understands how the ED works, s/he will never again argue with an ED nurse when they call the ICU stating they have to admit a patient immediately due to others coming in the door. The most helpful strategy for conflict resolution that I have used involves refocusing team members on the shared group goal(s). Ask what's best for the patient, and that will usually get discussion flowing in the right direction again. Team members tend not to argue when the focus is on patient outcomes.

 **For your toolkit…Keep the focus is on patient outcomes**

It is important to remind the team members of their commitment to the group during a conflict management stage. Take some time to define each team member's responsibility to meeting stated goals of the unit or group. Define the expected outcomes and timeframe for achieving them. Be sure to re-visit conflict resolution if a team member is not willing or not able to meet their team responsibilities. Have the team re-visit the goals and expected outcomes of care on a regular basis to ensure that the quality improvement process is inherent in daily practice.

Team conflict can also be triggered by transition and change. Change makes many people uncomfortable. Change involves letting go of old practices and expectations, but can also mean doing your job more effectively. Change often causes fear, grief and loss. Some people adapt better to change than others. People are like popcorn and "pop" (adapt) to change and new ideas at different times.

Because bedside care management is mandatory in today's healthcare environment, a team approach is necessary to for that to occur. Care management is critical to achieve positive patient outcomes and a perfect fit for both the patient and the team approach. Bedside care management enhances physician, payer, patients' and clinician satisfaction. It is a different concept that focusing team member efforts on daily tasks. Team members must remember to incorporate tasks within the entire patient perspective and care planning. Keep the perspective of the "total patient"; not just "tasks". "Tasks" are not all that healthcare workers do, although performance of tasks within the scope of practice is inherent in job responsibilities each day.

Bedside care management improves utilization of resources, job satisfaction and decreases patient length of stay. A team approach means true care management for the patient.

Discussion Questions:
1. Define the role of a supervisor, identifying important traits and tasks.
2. Explain the difference between authoritarian and participative management styles, how they differ in the workplace, including results with both styles.
3. Discuss the concept of discipline as a supervisor.
4. List 6 unforgivable supervisory mistakes.
5. Explain the different management theories including theory X,Y,Z,C,T, comparing and contrasting each style in the healthcare workplace.

6. Identify 6 differences between managers and leaders and explain why you chose them.

7. Explain the process of decision making, both positive and negative methods,

8. Explain the process of problem solving, both positive and negative methods.

Case Study/Role Playing:

Opening statement: you have achieved a position of leadership in our health-care community. Could you tell me a bit about your background and the role you are in today?

1. How would you describe a leader?

2. What are important qualities or characteristics of a leader?

3. Explain your personal philosophy of leadership.

4. What learning experiences have had the most influence on your personal development as a leader?

5. How do you see leadership evolving in healthcare today?

6. What are the most challenging issues in your current positions? Why?

7. As a leader/manager in your career, have you had a mentor? If so, how did this impact your leadership style. If not, why did you not use a mentor and how did that affect your style?

8. What advice would you give someone aspiring to a leadership position?

YOUR EVOLVING CAREER

YOUR EVOLVING CAREER

Chapter Objectives:

1. Identify and explain the 5 usual functions of healthcare workers regardless of specialty.
2. Explain the difference between being a knowledge worker and a technical worker.
3. Explain the method of dealing with an angry patient or co-worker.
4. Identify assertive communication style and why it is effective.
5. List and explain the different types of power and why they are necessary in the healthcare workplace.
6. List 4 myths of use of power.
7. Explain conflict and identify issues related to experiencing it.

Key terms

Conflict management	dealing with angry staff or patients
Power myths	types of power
Assertive style	knowledge vs. technical worker

Professional Healthcare Roles

The healthcare professional fulfills specific functions within their specific scope of practice specialty. It is important to know what those functions include when evaluating and enhancing your career. There are five usual functions of a healthcare worker, no matter what the specialty or role is. These functions include:

- Care provider– demonstrates skills in specific specialty, communication skills

- Teacher– demonstrates knowledge of basic principles of the teaching-learning process. Identifies clients' learning needs, capabilities and limitations, selection of appropriate information, material and strategies.

- Advocate– can state clients' rights and responsibilities as healthcare consumers, and identifies any issues between the clients and provider's perceptions of healthcare needs. May participates in client care conferences communicating clients' needs.

- Professional– demonstrated knowledge of the standards/criteria of competent performance and scope of professional specialty practice. Access own capabilities, limitations and accept accountability for actions. Establish goals for achieving professional growth.

- Supervisor– coordinate care of clients' to achieve care outcomes and the provision of cost-effective, quality based services.

(*adapted from American Association of Colleges of Nursing 5 roles of nursing, 1998)

Each healthcare professional fulfills these functions in the professional practice setting. It doesn't matter whether you work in a hospital, home health agency, school or church. You perform these functions every day. Assess your skills and abilities in each role. What are you best at doing? Why? Which of these roles are challenges for you? Why? This will help you evaluate the skills and competencies you need to enhance and expand.

There are other additional functions that every healthcare worker must exhibit in the workplace to be successful. The additional functions I have identified that each healthcare worker needs to develop include being a knowledge worker, not just a technical worker. Assist your healthcare facility to achieve organizational success. Be a participant in changing the healthcare organizational culture as well as your personal headspace. If you are a registered nurse, you must act as the care choreographer for patients. All healthcare workers, can active in managing your own personal transition as well as organizational transition. Talk with your colleagues and friends, and use them to validate your own professional malaise issues and behaviors. Demonstrating these kinds of behaviors will allow you to become indispensable at work.

Being indispensable is easier than it sounds. While there are deepening healthcare specialty shortages in some fields, there are still ways to make your self stand out in your current job setting. Focus your time on enhancing your skills, improving competencies and cultivating new ones. You will improve daily and have experiences that prepare you for new and different roles in the future. As you are working on honing your skills, you will also encounter situations that are challenging to handle, such as angry patients or co-workers.

Dealing with Angry Patients and Coworkers

If you are confronted by an angry co-worker in a work setting what should you do? It is crucial to resist the impulse to get angry. Be quiet and listen to the co-worker. Upset people want to be heard more than anything else. Try not to plan what you are going to say back to them while they are talking. This interferes with your ability to listen. Don't jump in and answer right away; wait until they stop talking. Wait silently for a few seconds before you respond. Resist the urge to tell them that they shouldn't feel the way they do. Feelings are valid even when you don't agree. If you have made a mistake, acknowledge that you have done so, and apologize.

 **For your toolkit....Remember, Upset people want to be heard. Wait until they stop talking to respond calmly.**

Other anger management strategies include trying to dispel false beliefs about the situation. Many times, anger is based on misperceptions and miscommunications. Wait until you are both calm to talk about the situation. You can then explain the situation the way you perceive it. This often goes a long way to dispel misperceptions. It is appropriate to recognize feel, express and accept your own anger. Try not to speak while you are angry, as you are likely to make impulsive and unkind comments.

Talk to a friend about the situation and your feelings. Sometimes it helps to role play an interaction with a trusted colleague or friend before you meet with the co-worker. You can also use physical activity to dispel your anger.

You can also try venting your anger to an inanimate object if there is no one to talk with.

Assertive Communication

Assertive communication is another important career strategy to master. Assertive communication is used for making and refusing requests, giving and receiving recognition and giving and receiving criticism (2012) Samples of an assertive communication style are those that describe the situation or behavior e.g. "when you…." and expresses your reactions or feelings about it "I feel…" You would also use an assertive style to specify the change that you want to occur, e.g. "I want you to…" Assertive style also allows you to identify common goals or outcomes, e.g. "if that happens, then…." or "if you do this, then…."

It is common to have some anxiety and fear when considering use of an assertive style of communication. If you are anxious or fearful of this, use relaxation techniques to help you prepare. Avoid self-defeating thoughts about how you think the communication exchange will occur. Use desensitization to break your fear into smaller steps to handle them. Visualization and guided imagery may also help you focus your approach. Ask for coaching from a trusted colleague or mentor and provide your own self-coaching by being patient with your anxiety.

Using Power for Managing Conflict

Power is one of the most important job skills you can utilize. Power is not necessarily related to a position in an organization. When you have power and use it well, you can influence many events and processes in your workplace. Power is defined as the ability to control, influence or act. Authority is defined as the legitimate power granted to an individual by an organization. Power is vested in a position. Leadership is the relationship between two or more people in which one influences the other toward accomplishing a goal without legitimate power. (Bernard and Walsh, 1996)

 **For your toolkit... When you use power well, you can influence many events and processes in your workplace.**

There are several different types of power, as defined in management texts. Personal power is the ability to link the outer capacity for action with the inner capacity of reflection. Organizational power is the ability to accomplish goals through others within an organization. Executive power is the use of personal persuasion and influence to motivate others.

Legitimate power is given to individuals based on their position in an organization. Reward power is the power to provide distribution of rewards. Coercive power is the ability to administer punishment, or the opposite of reward. Expert power is earned by an individual with expert knowledge and skills in a certain area or industry. Referent power is the ability to have influence over another based on respect and admiration.

Managers need both power (all of the types) and authority to be effective. Healthcare workers often see power as bad or negative, but it is actually a neutral force. People who tend to feel powerless often display the inability to accomplish a goal. Powerless people often resort to other methods to get what they want, such as manipulation, dishonesty and illegal behaviors. People with power move through different management states of being with their power, beginning with dictatorship. Some individuals never move past a dictator state. Others move through power states to seduction, persuasion, role modeling and finally to empowerment.

There are several myths about power. These include:

MYTH	*REALITY*
Power is bad	Power is neutral
Power is a goal	Power is a means to accomplish goals
Powerful people are ruthless	Powerless people are ruthless
Power can be given to others	Power must be earned or assumed

| It is wrong or bad to want power | Power to accomplish goals can reduce stress and frustration |

Power becomes very important in carrying out management and leadership activities. Strong leaders use all forms of power every day to accomplish goals and motivate people in their oversight to assist in meeting those goals. The use of power also may cause conflict.

Conflict is inevitable in life and at work due to complex organizations, differing employee interests and needs, and change related to transition. Many healthcare workers are not comfortable with conflict because they have had no training to deal with it. Healthcare education programs do not provide much training in conflict management or conflict resolution skills.

Conflict can make individuals and groups feel scared and powerless. Union organizers often point out how employees may feel powerless unless they are represented by a union– whether or not the employees are actually powerless. Like power, conflict is not bad. It is inherently neutral. Conflict is not personal. But people often make it into a personal situation. Conflict can be functional because it leads to discussion, investigation and accomplishment of new goals. Excessive conflict can be dysfunctional and leads to more strife, not problem solving.

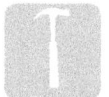 **For your toolkit....Conflict is not bad or personal; it is inherently neutral.**

Dysfunction organizations usually have lots of unresolved conflict. The senior management team may not be comfortable working through conflict to create new goals and priorities. Usually, dysfunctional organizations have a minimal amount of one way communication-from the top down. Failing to follow through on tasks, not giving positive reinforcement to managers and staff will add to perceptions of conflict. A leadership team that does not respect its' members, deal with conflict constructively or utilize effective communication, is creating a dysfunctional organization.

Before resolution of conflict can begin, the cause of the conflict must be identified. There are different types of conflict. There is conflict within a person or a group, between groups, or between organizations. There are different causes of conflict at work, including goal incompatibility, competition for scarce resources, task interdependencies, such as work shared between departments, organizational structure, and integration of roles. Groups are a frequent source of conflict because people come with their own set of values, history, and expectations. Ethnic and cultural diversity of the healthcare work force can also lead to conflict, as well as differing communication styles.

From my perspective as a consultant, conflict is over-feared and under-valued. Conflict happens every day to each of us. It is a part of life-from the moment we wake up in the morning. We experience and handle many different types of conflict. When I had my carpet cleaned recently, the man from the cleaning company arrived late and was rude and unfriendly. When he entered my house, he asked me why I was wasting my money cleaning such old and ugly carpet. This was not a great way to start off our encounter! Sometimes supervisors use work scheduling tactics that cause conflict for employees. Scheduling you on days you attend school or when you don't have day care undoubtedly will cause friction. The source of the conflict can't always be removed, but how you handle it is crucial to resolution. Many healthcare workers are ineffective in managing conflict.

 ## For your toolkit... Conflict is over-feared and under-valued.

Why is it that healthcare workers become ineffective when confronted with conflict in the workplace? Most healthcare workers would rather avoid conflict altogether than deal with whatever issue causes the tension. I'm not sure what makes conflict so difficult for healthcare workers. It may be lack of training in managing conflict. For some, undoubtedly, fear of the conflict resolution process is the hard part. For others, conflict may always be seen as a negative personal issue and therefore avoided at all costs. For the healthcare profession as a whole, conflict has often been avoided or glossed over and not dealt with. This has caused many formidable and difficult issues to be endlessly debated but never resolved.

Consider the touchy and sensitive topic of appropriate registered nursing educational preparations. Discussion has been going on over whether entry into nursing practice should be at the associate degree or baccalaureate level for at least forty years, and there is still no defined entry into practice education statement for all of nursing. Various professional organizations and states have created their own statements, but no universal set of expectations has yet been created.

According to Bernard and Walsh, (1996) conflict is a normal, unavoidable part of human relationships and can be a growth producing process if people learn how to manage it effectively. From the perspective of Hitt et al, (1986) although each conflict situation has unique causes, most can be traced to four major sources: goal incompatibility, competition for scarce resources, task interdependencies and organizational structure.

Consider this situation. You are working in a Diagnostic Imaging Department as a manager, and the CEO tells you at a management meeting that he has invited all the physicians from a neighboring hospital to start using your department for their emergency patients. You are already short-staffed and do not have enough help for emergent patients because there are already scheduled outpatients waiting for procedures on top of the admitted patients and your hospital emergency patients. How excited will you be to have more patients in your department? This is a great example of goal incompatibility.

If you are short of healthcare workers and count on the staffing office of your unit to provide you with employees, what happens when six units each want a different healthcare worker, and there are only four healthcare workers scheduled? This becomes a conflict over scarce resources. If you work in the intensive care unit on the night shift, and the Admitting department determines that they will no longer staff an admissions clerk on the night shift, you are affected by that decision. If the admissions manager makes that decision without talking to the ICU manager, and the nurses in ICU are expected to create admission documents on all new admits to ICU, you will have a conflict over task interdependencies. If you are a manager called to an emergency management meeting at 4:00 p.m. on a Friday afternoon and the CEO doesn't show up because he is leaving on a trip with his family, you will likely feel conflict over the organizational structure and lack of respect in your facility.

Conflict exists when two or more parties (individuals, groups or organizations) differ with regard to facts, opinions, beliefs, feelings, drives, needs, goals, methods, values or anything else. (Bernard and Walsh, 1996) The conflict produced by the differences between these parties creates tension and discomfort. Because of the discomfort conflict causes, most people view conflict as negative and something to be avoided if possible. There are managers and executives who perceive that shouting at a subordinate is the way to solve conflict. This is not the case, and beside that, is highly unprofessional. I have a colleague who recently told me that she cannot remember the last time she and her boss (a vice president) had a calm discussion about what they disagreed on. Her boss yells at her whenever they disagree. Not only is that approach extremely unprofessional, it is a huge staff retention issue!

I encountered a boss a few years ago who thought it was a good idea to use profanity to get his point across. While I wasn't personally offended, it put off lots of people who were so focused on his use of "bad language" that they didn't hear what he actually said. It is also likely that he could have made all the points he wanted without using language that makes some people uncomfortable.

Disagreement between groups about their goals can create conflict, especially if the accomplishment of one group's goals prevents the other group from achieving its goals. If a hospital wants to change how units are staffed and a healthcare worker bargaining unit from a labor union files a grievance, the union group can inhibit the achievement of the reconstructed staffing. This becomes incredibly frustrating for everyone involved, even when the objections to a new strategy are valid. Consider something like electronic medical records. If you see benefits for you in not implementing electronic medical records technology, then you will feel conflict if your unit is to transition into an electronic medical record charting system. Competition for scarce resources is an all-too-common theme for conflict in today's healthcare institutions. Dollars, people, space and time are all in short supply.

If you depend on another unit or department to help you achieve your goals, conflict will occur if that department achieves a goal that negatively affects your department. As in the previous example, closing the Admitting office after midnight may be seen as a great cost saving measure by the Admitting department, but as a major inconvenience for the ER or ICU night shift staff.

Most organizational structures also cause conflict to occur. Differing goals, roles and viewpoints between managers and subordinates, or project managers and operations staff, are common and often difficult to resolve. In this era of constantly increasing healthcare costs and ever-decreasing health care dollars, there is more conflict than ever!

Some healthcare workers may be unprepared to handle conflict. Many healthcare workers are women and in some cultures, women may not be brought up to deal with conflict. While this is not universally true, men tend to be socialized to see conflict as a usual occurrence in life, not as a personal attach or unusual situation. This may be partially due to men having more exposure to competitive sports, where conflict reigns on the field, but friendships endure once the game is over.

The other challenge for healthcare workers in dealing with conflict situations is the issue of accountability. Sometimes healthcare workers perceive they have no personal accountability for affecting change to a situation based on something they believe in. This may be due to perceiving themselves as not having any decision making power as a staff worker or expecting someone else to handle the problem. Many patient care improvements have been initiated because staff workers decided to change some aspect of care they felt strongly about. Family at the bedside during a code blue or creating blood sugar management protocols in a critical care unit are examples of healthcare workers effectively managing conflict to affect a positive change.

Change almost always causes conflict. Conflict is part off the natural change process. Although individuals can be resistant to the current changes we are seeing in healthcare, the impetus for change is coming from both outside (e.g. the federal government) and inside the healthcare industry. Conflict results from implementing changes such as insurance-covered well baby care or pain management documentation requirements or new quality initiatives created by federal agencies. Conflict can resolve differences, clarify issues, and promote unity when managed effectively. To avoid conflict is to eliminate the possibility of defining goals, discussing issues, and designing a unifying philosophy about the issue.

 **For your toolkit... Conflict is part off the natural change process.**

Conflict can also be about power. If you are a leader who implements change, conflict will inevitably result as a by-product of that change. For a leader to use his/her power effectively, s/he must deal with the conflict in order for the change process to take place. To avoid conflict is to ignore the power of leadership. Surrendering power creates ineffective leaders and limits change potential when health care organizations constantly need it.

Conflict in and of itself is not bad. It creates tension and makes people feel uncomfortable. Ignoring conflict and tension is what causes poor problem resolution, frustration and defensiveness. Conflict is often seen as negative. The negativity is not inherent in conflict itself, but rather comes from tension caused by not handling the original issue or because of inappropriate methods of dealing with the issue (remember the screaming VP or the guy that swears). Healthcare workers often fear conflict because the tension it creates makes them less articulate and the increased stress, workload and time demands make any conflict feel personal.

Conflict does enhance advocacy. Above all else, healthcare workers continually strive to be advocates. Patients, families and the under-served are the recipients of that advocacy. Handling conflict effectively allows patient advocacy to flourish. To not deal with conflict limits patient advocacy and intervention effectiveness.

There are two ways to deal with conflict. One way is to utilize conflict resolution. There are different types of conflict resolution techniques, including team building, sharing perspectives non-defensively, attempting to focus on cooperative goals, transition management, education and communication. Conflict resolution seeks a solution that completely satisfies all parties involved in the conflict. Rarely is it possible to satisfy all the needs of everyone involved. Some compromises are usually made by all parties to reach agreement. Legal arbitration is a type of conflict resolution.

The more common way to deal with conflict is through conflict management, which implies a conscious effort to deal with the conflict as well as the issue and control the problem. It does not guarantee to satisfy all involved, but attempts to meet as many needs as possible in determining a solution. (Bernard and Walsh, 1996)

There are numerous issues that enter into a conflict situation. The values, goals, resources, and beliefs of the people involved will affect their willingness to compromise and resolve the issues. Past relationships between conflicting parties are also important. If you have no respect for or do not trust your adversary, chances are you will not be committed to managing the conflict.

Healthcare workers apply different strategies to conflict situations. The first choice is often to deny that the conflict exists. This causes no change in the conflict situation at all. If denial doesn't work, some healthcare workers try to ignore conflict. This may relieve the tension initially, but the relief is usually short-lived. Ignoring conflict causes relationships to further deteriorate and people will keep feeling bad. Suppressing conflict may be why people think of it as negative and destructive.

While difficult, it is much easier in the long run to deal with conflict head on. Confrontation means letting the other party know you disagree and being willing to discuss the issues using collaboration, arbitration, problem solving or compromise. Many healthcare workers who deal with conflict get stuck in the confrontation and never get to the discussion phase.

Not dealing with conflict is the single most limiting factor in resolving healthcare issues at both the local and national levels. The nursing profession in particular has yet to be comfortable with the ideas that conflict is a valuable process and creative dissonance is beneficial to addressing changing issues. Instead of dealing with conflict up front, nursing groups tend to "take sides" according to special interests. No formal confrontation takes place, and as a result, the profession is perceived as divisive and splintered in its beliefs and goals.

Physicians are usually more comfortable dealing with conflict than other healthcare workers. They certainly have just as many issues to disagree on, but physicians are usually able to "duke it out" behind closed doors and come out with a united stance for their profession. I remember being in an interdisciplinary hospital meeting with both physicians and healthcare workers on the committee. Two physicians got into a yelling match over a specific patient protocol. They argued most of the meeting. When the meeting was over and they were walking out the door, they were discussing their next opportunity to meet for a golf game. Clearly, their conflict was not personalized and did not encroach on their personal relationship.

Healthcare workers could learn from that approach. We could be so much more powerful in dealing with healthcare social policy issues if the professionals were willing to "get down and dirty" to resolve its differences before airing its dirty laundry and splintered decisions in public. As a profession, nursing tends to look like the right hand doesn't know what the left hand is doing when it comes to important intra-professional issues like educational entry into practice, instead of arbitrating our conflicts about resolution and drawing a unified stance to share with patients and the public.

The formation of the Federal Nursing Commission for the Institute of Medicine Study on Nursing Staff in Hospitals and Nursing Homes is a classic example of not dealing with conflict and going public with the issues before discussion. Chances are no commission would have been needed and almost 1 million dollars in federal funds could have been saved if nursing representatives could have dealt with the perceptions and conflicts over staffing, patient care outcomes and nursing injuries before hand. I had the privilege of providing testimony at the hearings on this topic, and heard the chairman share a similar perspective about the formation of the commission.

Conflict will always have to co-exist with healthcare. Healthcare staff will continue to disagree on issues fundamental to their profession and critical to patient advocacy. Resolving conflict takes a strong stomach and the willingness to be uncomfortable. Healthcare workers need to learn to see that differing opinions are not unusual or bad and that dissonance fosters creativity, innovation and collaborative outcomes. Healthcare workers need to stop being afraid of conflict and start learning to use it.

Discussion Questions:

1. Explain the 5 usual functions of healthcare workers regardless of specialty, and provide an example of each in your specialty.

2. Explain the difference between being a knowledge worker and a technical worker. Why does it matter?

3. Demonstrate a method of dealing with an angry patient or co-worker.

4. Identify/role play assertive communication style and why it is effective. Samples of an assertive communication style are those that describe the situation or behavior e.g. "when you...." and expresses your reactions or feelings about it "I feel..." You would also use an assertive style to specify the change that you want to occur, e.g. "I want you to..." Assertive style also allows you to identify common goals or outcomes, e.g. "if that happens, then...." or "if you do this, then...."

5. Explain the different types of power and why they are necessary in the healthcare workplace.

6. Explain the concept of power and list 4 myths and realities when using power.

7. Explain conflict and identify issues related to experiencing it.

8. Discuss and explain an issue causing conflict within your healthcare specialty and potential resolution ideas.

Case Studies:

1. Sarah was a new manager in a community hospital. She had been in her role less than a year. A physician came up to her, clearly upset, and started screaming at her about a patient whose lab work was not yet in the chart for his review. How should Sarah respond to the MD? Why?

2. Betsy was a chief nurse executive of a large healthcare organization. She routinely told half truths or untruths to her staff. She made a point of critiquing leadership styles of her staff in public locations. She routinely sat with the CEO of the organization. You are a staff member who works for Betsy. What should you about her, if anything?

CREATING YOUR HEALTHCARE FUTURE

A "turned-on person" has a vision of self and knows who they are, has abundant energy and helps others discover their identity"
-Author unknown

FUTURE TRENDS IN HEALTHCARE

Chapter 11 Objectives:

1. Identify 3 future trends in healthcare and how they will affect your specialty.
2. List two environmental factors that impact your healthcare practice and specialty.
3. List the goals of the triple aim initiative.
4. Identify the components of the healthcare framework in the future.
5. Define and explain an ACO.

Key terms

Triple aim initiative
diversity
aging
technology
workforce
healthcare financing
healthcare structures

Medicare
ACO
healthcare framework
self-governance
healthcare architecture
retention

Future Trends in Healthcare

One of my favorite quotes was in healthcare magazine years ago from the managed care guru Paul Gann. "It is easy to come up with new ideas; the hard part is letting go of what worked for you two years ago, but will soon be out of date." It has never been truer for healthcare practices than right now at the early part of a new millennium.

In the past, the architecture of healthcare has been based on a foundation of patient advocacy and achieving maximum beneficial outcomes for each patient. The framework of care for patients included specialization of services, fragmented components of care, a narrow focus with minimum flexibility and an "us vs. them" mentality. Some professions, such as nursing has taken direction from other professions in terms of work tasks. Nurses have allowed other disciplines to dictate their scope of practice and role. Nurses have redesigned their role around other healthcare staff, such as Clinical Dieticians, Respiratory Therapists, Physical Therapists, and Occupational Therapists. This framework is no longer compatible with the direction of the healthcare industry. Every specialty has defined roles and behaviors that have evolved in the new healthcare environment.

Several environmental factors are impacting the future of healthcare practice. These factors include:

1. Diversity–changing demographics in states' populations, the diversity of the healthcare workforce and public views of healthcare and healthcare policy issues.

2. Aging–impact of an aging population on healthcare systems, financing of healthcare and demand for some healthcare professions (nursing, pharmacists, dental hygienists) aging nursing workforce, and the development of new healthcare services.

3. Technology–the impact of global technology on healthcare roles and practice .

4. Workforce–challenges in healthcare workforce supply, demand, education and role definition.

5. Healthcare financing–increasing costs and financing impact on delivery systems, community based health programs and healthcare practice roles.

6. New structures– required to meet future needs e.g. Accountable Care Organizations, part of the Obama Healthcare Reform Act currently under review in the Supreme Court. Accountable Care Organizations (ACOs) are groups of doctors, hospitals, and other health care providers, who come together voluntarily to give coordinated high quality care to their Medicare patients.

To meet the needs of our nation for the future, the healthcare professions must be part of the changing framework in which care is provided. The architectural foundation remains the same. Patient advocacy and maximum beneficial care outcomes will continue to drive the way care is provided. However, we must eliminate much of the intra-professional infighting and competition between professional roles that has kept us from achieving our goals and finding ways to fundamentally affect the health of our nation.

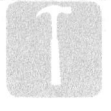 **For your toolkit... The healthcare professions must change the framework in which care is provided.**

The framework that healthcare must build for future practice must be focused on specific professional roles as well as integration of services, a community wide focus, flexibility and cross training of staff, commitment to life-long learning and professional development, the mindset of "us helping them" and one focused, professional voice with which care practices are changed to meet the needs of all patients.

Accountable Care Organizations are designed to provide consistent care of high quality to a specific group of patients while controlling costs. According to the Institute of Medicine, there were many poor patient outcomes that could be prevented (Crossing the Quality Chasm, 2001). In 2007, work continued and a report by the Institute of Healthcare Improvement launched the Triple Aim Initiative (2007). This initiative was designed to:

- Improve the health of the population
- Enhance patients' experience of care including quality, access and reliability
- Control or reduce cost of care

To evaluate how to achieve this, certain existing high performance healthcare delivery organizations were studied. These systems utilized information continuity, patient engagement, care coordination, team-oriented care delivery, continuous innovation and convenient access to care (2010). These studies and reports were incorporated into the healthcare act of 2010. This new law offers financial incentives for healthcare entities to become ACOs (2010).

ACOs are a dramatic change for current healthcare delivery. The hope is that ACOs can overcome the fragmentation and volume based processes of the fee for service system, to eliminate providers getting paid based on the number of tests and procedures ordered. It is also a possibility that ACOs can shift healthcare from a focus on illness and injury to a focus of health and wellness. Hospitals, skilled nursing, long-term acute care, hospice and mental health facilities can all be part of ACOs as well as physicians, independent practitioners and outpatient facilities. ACOs are a terrific opportunity for independent practitioners such as advanced practice nurses, physical therapists, psychologists, social workers and alternative medicine specialties to get involved in a wellness-based structure for healthcare delivery.

To achieve this new architecture and framework for healthcare practice, there are additional changes that will be seen across the profession within the next 20 years. We need to expect exponential change and an accelerated rate of change compared to the past decades. Healthcare education, especially nursing and pharmacy programs, will be vastly different. Students will take core courses online. Healthcare education programs will utilize multi-media and on-site clinical experiences like human simulation labs. An internship at the end of school and a residency at the beginning of the new graduates' first year will be required.

Healthcare providers will be everywhere-affecting health in every feasible location—churches, schools, homeowners associations, shopping malls. They will be seen as chronic care coaches and managers. Patients will see physicians only when their conditions change. Nurses will be perceived as highly skilled, caring, and well educated professionals. Through the roles of clinician, coach, educator and entrepreneur, the handmaiden image of the traditional nurse will finally die.

Healthcare professionals will be multi-culturally competent with additional advance practice skills such as leadership, educator, and supervisor. They will be information gurus and spend much of their time harnessing and explaining information to others. Because of these enhanced roles, and the continued nursing shortage in spite of the poor economy, the demand for healthcare workers, personal care aides and unlicensed assistive personnel will continue to rise. Over half of the fastest growing occupations are in healthcare roles (BLS, 2/ 1/ 2012).

The healthcare workplace will be transformed. Staggered and part time shifts will be the norm. Roles like Retention Coordinator and Master Preceptor will be created for older and very experienced professionals. Clinical staff will be faculty in local healthcare programs and schools. Patient care will be monitored from nurses' homes. Robots will be used to provide care in remote location, directed by a clinician in an urban setting. There will be no paper, no needles, with searchable electronic medical records and patient histories available throughout the US.

Retention will be the healthcare focus instead of recruitment, especially as boomers retire. The priority will shift to keeping staff in the workforce, especially the "boomer nurses and pharmacists." New retention strategies will be identified and implemented using "out of the box" thinking. Significant pension plans, paid education sabbaticals and extended vacation time will be the norm.

Scheduling will be "cafeteria style" where staff can pick what works best for them. Positions will be thought of in terms of a commitment of worked hours per pay period or month, and staff can pick a plan that works for them. Self-scheduling will be the norm, and salaries will reflect weekend and holiday commitments.

There are some challenges to this kind of optimal professionalization and self-determination of healthcare practice. These challenges include regulation of healthcare practice by organizations juxtaposed with the self-directed autonomy of healthcare practice. Unionization of professional staff versus self-governance of staff will become a hot debate by the end of this current decade. There will likely be less union workers in healthcare, as professional workers realize autonomy and shared governance work better than militancy and an "us vs. them mentality", particularly in a tepid economy. There will be a wide diversity of healthcare values that may overshadow shared beliefs and collaborative strategies for the healthcare professions.

There will continue to be intra-professional practice conflicts related to good boundary management of what belongs in nursing practice and what is and what is not the realm of other practitioners. There will be more focused dialog on education differentiation in nursing (ADN,BSN and MSN) and agreement on what the minimum educational foundation for all professional practice should be. This will likely be ongoing dialog with practice changes over many years. There will be defined roles for alternative healthcare specialties, intertwined with traditional roles.

The preferred future for healthcare will require specific leadership strategies. These strategies will include autonomy for professional practice and career development and a knowledge-based foundation for practice. Healthcare staff will develop leadership skills and competencies and work intensively to improve the public perception of their professions. The utilization of evidenced based practice, outcomes focused measurements for patients, and research based practice will be commonplace.

Most healthcare professions will work in a self-governed workforce in a shared governance model within healthcare organizations. Labor unions will have less impact on staffing ratios and utilization because these items will be determined by the professions themselves. There will be minimal regulations with regard to staffing and other professional practice issues, as individual professions will set their own criteria well above current regulatory standards. This will require both professional and workplace points of influence on healthcare practice. There will be social and community activism around health and policy related issues. All of these strategies will mandate the creation of a lifelong learning environment for healthcare professionals.

The role of the registered nurse in the future will be as a director and coordinator of care, not just a task provider. Nurses will become the choreographer of care for patients. Other professions will support the care delivery continuum. Many healthcare roles will have an expanded practice with a redirected focus towards wellness. They will function in a community-based model using a case management approach to care along the health-illness continuum. Front line healthcare staff will continue routinely recognized as the work task redesign experts. They will maintain basic skills and core competencies.

All these changes will require great transition management skills. Healthcare professionals will need to create strategies for "making the incredible credible and the impossible possible", according to Richard Brock RN, MN. Acknowledge your uniqueness and revel in keeping that intact. Don't try to cope alone and use your circle of support – friends, spouse, significant others, colleagues. This will help you manage your stress. Remember what your mother told you, but thrive on how things are changing so you can survive!

Creating your Personal Healthcare Future

Only you can determine the kind of healthcare professional you want to be. It is easy to be passionate about a profession that gives you so many job options and career choices. Healthcare forces you to be the best you can be, no matter what your role. It is difficult for the general public to grasp that other healthcare professions, like nurses and alternative medicine practitioners–not physicians–are rapidly becoming the fulcrum of healthcare with the Obama Healthcare Reform Act. The nursing, pharmacist and other professional shortages have further escalated the problems of a broken healthcare system.

Life-long learning throughout your healthcare career will put you on the path to excellence. Life is about learning, and learning is about change. You must do both to carve out your personal future in healthcare. If you lack awareness of changing circumstances or an attitude that embraces change, your professional growth will be stunted. Life-long learning complements the professional growth that comes with self-conscious experience. (DiLeonardi, 2005) Healthcare professionals committed to lifelong learning for their own professional development will have an exciting future!

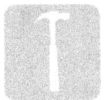 **For your toolkit... Life is about learning, and learning is about change.**

According to Susan Gordon, those of us in healthcare and particularly nursing, have the power to make or break healthcare right now–and for years to come. (2005) Each one of us has a responsibility as a professional to secure care for our nation's population as well our specialty profession's future. We hold the keys to the solutions to change systems and processes. Be sure you use your influence to enhance care and your profession in a positive way.

Using your healthcare influence to enhance care is really about being a leader in society and using leadership skills. Dr. Warren Bennis is an internationally recognized management and leadership guru. At the time, as the Chairman of the Leadership Institute at the University of Southern California, he defined leadership in one sentence. "A leader is one who manifests direction integrity, hardiness and courage in a consistent pattern of behavior that inspires trust, motivation and responsibility on the part of the followers who in turn become leaders themselves."(1998)

Bennis goes onto say that there are four basic competencies of leaders that are inherent in that definition. I believe healthcare professionals have all of them. Bennis believes that people want four things from their leaders. "First, direction and meaning; second, trust; third, a sense of hope and optimism—some way of investing in the future; and finally, they want results. These are the four things that all people want." (1998) Leaders have to provide a sense of purpose to give direction and meaning. They have to be authentic to provide trust. They have to enable and develop authentic relationships, and they have to have a sense of hardiness in order to provide that sense of optimism and hope.

Leaders are people that generally believe things will work out well and that one can influence the circumstances of one's life-an expectation for success. Leaders also have a bias toward action, as well as courage and the ability to act. Effective leaders, given the original definition from Bennis, have to actually provide purpose, enable authentic relationships among people, have a sense of hardiness themselves, and have the courage to take risks and act. This describes most healthcare roles in a nutshell. Most healthcare staff I have known possess these characteristics inside their souls.

Use your own healthcare soul every day, whatever role you are in. Generate a sense of purpose in your organization that honors your profession and the patients you care for. Spread your vision and purpose throughout the institution and give fellow colleagues a sense of meaning. Keep reminding people what is important. Encourage people to be straightforward and honest. This will encourage healthy discussion and resistance. Leadership is really about being empathic and caring about whom people really are. Leadership is being candid all the time and "walking the talk". Given the complexity of life and healthcare, leaders have to take decisive action as well as take some risks.

Many healthcare professionals are leaders. They are also winners at what they set out to accomplish. Start leading and exhibiting behaviors of a winner as soon as you finish this book. Healthcare is a career for life and a way of life. Support the renaissance of healthcare professions by mentoring kindly those who come after you, and showing them the ways of the future. Demonstrate the qualities of a winner as you plan your career goals and your future. Good luck!

Discussion Questions:

1. Identify 3 future trends in healthcare and discuss how they will affect different healthcare specialties.
2. Discuss environmental factors that impact your healthcare practice and specialty.
3. Discuss whether the Triple Intiative is a good idea and why.
4. Discuss the environmental factors' effects on healthcare and determine potential ramifications.
5. Discuss the new healthcare framework for the future.
6. Discuss the effect of ACOs in your geographic area.
7. Discuss what Warren Bennis believes people want from their leaders.

Case Studies:

1. Henry is a hospital CEO. He is the CEO of the biggest hospital in a small healthcare system. He is well respected and enjoys the popularity that comes with working at a facility for 25 years in both clinical and administrative roles. He has been the CEO for 15 years. His qualities include finance skills, "clinical mindset", a strong relationship with board members and strong community relationships. His leadership style and characteristics include micromanagement, need to approve every document prior to it being sent by every manager,

lack of trust in key players, changing strategic direction frequently. Will he be successful in the next ten years? Why or why not?

2. You are asked by your boss to spearhead the development of an ACO in your community. Who will you meet with? Who are your stakeholders? Why? What steps will you take to set up this group?

THE WINNER

The Winner is always a part of the answer.
The Loser is always a part of the problem.
The Winner always has a program.
The Loser always has an excuse.
The Winner says, "Let me do it for you."
The Loser says "That's not my job"
The Winner sees an answer for every problem.
The Loser sees a problem for every answer.
The Winner says it may be difficult, but it's possible.
The loser says it may be possible, but it's too difficult.
A Winner listens.
A Loser waits until it's his turn to talk.
When a Winner makes a mistake, he says "I was wrong."
When a Loser makes a mistake, he says. "It wasn't my fault."
A Winner says "I'm good, but not as good as I could be."
A Loser says, "I'm not as lots of other people."
A Winner feels responsible for more than his job.
A Loser says "I only work here."

-Author unknown

HEALTHCARE CAREER GUIDE

REFERENCES

1. Association of California Nurse Leaders, *ACNL Resource Guide for Political Action*, 1995.
2. Cowles, Luke, "First Impressions", Advance for Nurses, March 7, 2005 p.23
3. Mehallow, Cindy, "Nursing Careers Beyond the Bedside"
4. http://featuredreports.monster.com/nursing05/nonclinical/
5. Mehallow, Cindy, "Nursing Careers Beyond the Hospital" http://featuredreports.monster.com/nursing05/nonhospital/
6. Rossheim, John "Nurses Who Teach"
7. http://featuredreports.monster.com/nursing05/professorship/
8. Malugani, Megan "Up-and-Coming Nurse Niches"
9. http://featuredreports.monster.com/nursing05/niches/
10. Malugani, Megan "Legal Nurse Consulting"
11. http://featuredreports.monster.com/nursing05/legal/
12. Meyeroff, Wendy J. "Advance Your Nursing Career"
13. http://featuredreports.monster.com/nursing05/advancedspecialties/
14. Worthington, Michael "Top 20 Recruiter Pet Peeves About Resumes", http://resumedoctor.com/
15. Gaffin, Norma Mushkat, "Recruiters' Top 10 Resume Pet Peeves"
16. http://resume.monster.com/articles/petpeeves/
17. Lipow, Valerie, "Interviewing 101" http://hourlyandskilled.monster.com/retail/articles/retailinterviewing/
18. Barada, Paul W. , "How Do You Sell Yourself When You Don't Have Much to Sell?" http://content.monstertrak.monster.com/resources/archive/jobhunt/toughsell/
19. Voght, Peter "Measure Your Soft Skills Smarts" http://content.monstertrak.monster.com/resources/archive/jobhunt/softskills

20. Advance News magazine, "Advancing Your Career" htto://www. advanceweb.com
21. Versant RN Residency www.versant.org
22. Smith, Mike, "Beyond Competent", Emergency Medical Services, June, 2005, pg 42.
23. Hollander, Jim. Onboard medical facilities have cruise passengers covered. *Los Angeles Times,* Sunday , June 26, 2005, pg L3
24. Buerhaus P., Implications of an Aging Registered Nurse Workforce *JAMA*, June 14, 2000; vol. 83, no. 22.
25. Dick, Thom, *Listening: Defusing the Angry Employee* Emergency Medical Services, June, 2005 p. 28
26. Rundio, Al *Ten management pearls for success"* Nurseweek, 2005
27. Pathways to success, p 24-5.
28. McLinden, Steve, *Navigating Organizational Culture,* Nurseweek, 2005
29. Pathways to success, p 102-05.
30. Gates, Polly Rubano, Joan; *Executive Coaching or Mentoring: Which way should you go?* DirectLink Newsletter, Association of California Nurse Leaders, Fall 2004,p.1
31. Brownstein, M. *Coaching and Mentoring for Dummies,* Foster City; IDE Books Worldwide, Ind. (2000)
32. Lewin, K. *Group decision and social change,* In Newcomb, T, Hartely E. ed., *Readings in Social Psychology,* New York, Holt, Rinehart Winston, 1947
33. Turner, Susan Odegaard, *Nurses guide to managed care,* 1999, Aspen Publishers
34. Turner, Susan Odegaard, *Has the Restructuring of Registered Nursing Roles in Hospitals Been Successful?* doctoral dissertation , College of Business, Southern California University, 1998
35. Turner, Susan Odegaard , *Transitions in Healthcare Series,* American Association of Critical Care Nurses, 1996
36. Stern, C. *Kaiser Foundation Hospital Graduate Nurse Handbook of Job Searching Techniques,* 4th ed, Oakland, California, Kaiser Permanente Hospitals (1990)

37. Kennedy, M. M. "When your career is sidelined" *Executive Female, September*/October, 1996. 33-35

38. yourownrubyslippers.com

39. the transitionnetwork.org

40. coachfederation.com

41. Advisory Board Daily Briefing (2001, April 9) "Severe Nursing Shortage is Threat to Patient Care",

42. Allen, Jane E (2001, May 7) "U.S. Nurses Not Alone in Their Frustration," Los Angeles Times.

43. Brown, Steve, (2001, May 21) "Congress Spotlights Nursing Shortage, Rural Wage Index Workforce Issues", AHA News 37(20).

44. Buerhaus, P., Staiger, D.O., and Auerbach, D.I., (2000). "Implications of an Aging Registered Nurse Workforce" Journal of the American Medical Association, 283 (22), 2948-2987.

45. Buerhaus P. (2000, June 14) "Implications of an Aging Registered Nurse Workforce." Journal of the American Medical Association, 83 (22).

46. California Board of Registered Nursing (2009), Annual School Report. Sacramento: author.

47. Coffman, J., Spetz, J., Seago, J.A., Rosenoff, E., O'Neil, E. (2001, January). Nursing in California: A Workforce Crisis. San Francisco: Workforce Initiative and the UCSF Center for the Health Professions.

48. Erwin J. (1999, March 29) "Aging Out? Will the Rising Age of O.R. Nurses Lead to a Shortage?" NurseWeek.

49. Fackelmann K. (2000, June 15) "Study Predicts Nursing Shortage" USA Today.

50. Hughes J. (2000, May 7) "Shortage in Profession Persists." Times Dispatch.

51. Russell G. (2000, April 21) "Nursing Schools See Enrollment Steadily Shrink", Telegram Gazette. RN Scope of Practice, California Business and Professional Code, Section 2725.

52. Ruiz M. (2000, Third Quarter) "Nursing Shortage" Sigma Theta Tau International Honor Society of Nursing in Clinical Practice. 2948-2954

53. "2000 National Sample Survey of Registered Nurses," Health Resources and Services Administration, author, .

54. Selis S. (2000, June) "Where Have All the Nurses Gone?" Healthcare Business. 3 (4), 65-70.

55. Buerhaus, Peter, changing demographics of nursing *Health Affairs* November

56. 17, 2004.

57. DeRitis, S. New Opportunities within Healthcare Informatics, *Advance,* April 26, 2004, p. 31.

58. Dr. Phil (McGraw) Column, Oprah, June 2005. p. 31.

59. Gladwell, Malcolm ,*Tipping Point*, Little Brown, New York,2004

60. Noer, David "After the Pink Slips" *Executive Female,* July/ August, 1995 p.43-45.

61. Kaye, B.L., Jordan-Evan, S. (2002). *Love 'em or lose 'em: Getting good people to stay.* San Francisco, CA. Benett-Koehler Publishers.

62. Abrams, M (2002, March). "Employee retention and turnover: Holding managers accountable" *Trustee.* Chicago, 55 (3), T1.

63. Hugg, Alicia, "Forging Ahead", *Nurseweek,* July 4, 2005, p.8-10.

64. Steefel, L. "Survey shows first real positive workforce change", *Nurseweek*, July 4, 2005 p.15.

65. Bach, David "Get that Raise" *Working Mother,* September 2005, p. 52.

66. Lichtenberg, Ronna "Designing a future that fits" *More* July/ August, 2005 p. 60-64.

67. Merritt, Jennifer, "Get-Ahead Strategies You've Never Heard Before" http:// reference.aol.com/onlinecampus/campusarticle?id=20050712200509990001

68. Thomas, D., 1994 "Five Ways to Run Your Career Like a business" *Executive Female*, November/December 37-40.

69. Hitt, M, Middlemist, R and Mathis, R, 1986, *Management concepts and effective practice,* 2nd ed. Houston, Texas, West Publishing.

70. Bernstein, A. and Craft-Rozen, S. "Why don't they just get it?" *Executive Female* March/April, 1995 p 33-7.

71. Beverly Health and Rehabilitation Services, Rancho Cordova, CA, *Supervisory Training Modules.*

72. Lyon, Mary "The ABCs of Pursuing Higher Education in Nursing", *Nurseweek Career Fair,* 1998.

73. Fischman, Josh **"Nursing Wounds",** *US News and World Report,* http://www.usnews.com/usnews/health/articles/020617/archive_021640.htm

74. Brzezicki, Lisa, "Caring for the Caregiver" *Advance for Nurses,* Southern California edition; August 22, 2005 p.9.

75. Mooney, Bette, "Resolving Conflicts" *Advance for Nurses,* Southern California edition, July 11,2005, p.15.

76. Bensing, K, "No Stone Unturned", *Advance for Nurses,* Southern California edition, August 8, 2005, p.11.

77. Goulette, Candy, "Under their Wings", *Advance for Nurses,* Southern California edition, June 13, 2005 p.38-9.

78. Johnson, James, "Warren Bennis, Chairman, The Leaderships Institute, *Healthcare Executive,* 1998 http://www.ache.org/pubs/hcexecsub.cfm

79. *Benefits of becoming a Magnet-designated facility* http://www.nursing-world.org/ancc/magnet/benes.html

80. Komisarjevskys, "Peanut Butter and Jelly Management: Tales from Parenthood Lessons for Managers" (Amacom, 2004).

81. Abrams, M (2002, March). Employee retention and turnover: Holding managers accountable. Trustee. Chicago, 55 (3), T1.

82. AONE. (2002, Sept.). Say what? What California nurses say about working, Nurseweek/AONE Study

83. Buckingham, M., Coffman, C. (~2001). First, break all the rules: What the world's greatest managers do differently. New York, NY. Simon & Schuster.

84. Robbins, Stephen, *Organizational behavior,* 7th ed. 1996, Prentice Hall.

85. Myss, Caroline, S*acred Contracts*, Three Rivers Press, New York, 2003

86. Stringer, Heather, "Turning Point" *Nurseweek*, August 29,2005, p. 12.

87. Deleonardi, Bette "Lifelong Learning," *Advance for Nurses,* September 5, 2005, p.17-22.

88. Warren, Rick *The Purpose Driven Life,* Zondervan, Michigan, 2002

89. https://www.cms.gov/Medicare/Medicare-Fee-for-Service-Payment/ACO/index.html?redirect=/ACO/.

90. http://www.bls.gov/emp/ep_table_103.htm

91. http://www.nhscareers.nhs.uk/atoz.shtml
92. http://www.bls.gov/oco/cg/cgs035.htm
93. http://explorehealthcareers.org/en/getting_started/is_a_health_ career_right
94. http://www.ama-assn.org/go/alliedhealth
95. http://www.aamc.org/students
96. http://bhpr.hrsa.gov/
97. http://www.caahep.org
98. http://www.bls.gov/ooh/
99. http://www.iom.edu/Reports/2001/Crossing-the-Quality-Chasm-A-New-Health-System-for-the-21st-Century.aspx
100. http://www.ihi.org/offerings/Initiatives/TripleAim/Pages/default.aspx
101. http://news.nurse.com/apps/pbcs.dll/article?AID=2012104230004
102. http://benefitsattorney.com/modules.php?name=Content&pa=showpag e&pid=14
103. http://www.personalbrandingblog.com/develop-your-career-like-a-business/
104. http://www.lifecoaching.com/pages/life_coaching.html
105. http://currentnursing.com/nursing_theory/Patricia_Benner_From_ Novice_to_Expert.html
106. http://entrepreneursuccesstools.com/2010/09/23/time-management-peter-drucker/
107. http://www.nwlink.com/~donclark/leader/leadcom.html ,2012
108. http://www.strategy-business.com/article/re00063?gko=ae079
109. Robbins, by Stephen P, Truth about managing people FT Press, 2 edition (September 30, 2007)
110. http://www.teamtechnology.co.uk/tuckman.html
111. Marks, Mitchell From Turmoil to Triumph: New Life After Mergers, Acquisitions, and Downsizing,1994
112. http://money.cnn.com/2011/07/27/pf/employee_pay/index.htm
113. http://www.compassionfatigue.org/
114. http://www.adldentallabs.com/dental/tech.htm
115. http://www.opcareers.org/

116. http://www.caahep.org/Content.aspx?ID=52
117. http://www.bls.gov/ooh/Healthcare/Physician-assistants.htm
118. http://www.mayoclinic.com/health/assertive/SR00042
119. http://managementhelp.org/personalproductivity/problem-solving.htm#guide
120. http://www.healthadministrationdegrees.com/articles/health-care-jobs/
121. http://www.nytimes.com/ hospitals/hiring/2008
122. http://www.healthcare.gov/law/full/index.html
123. http://www.healthcarejobs.org/education

www.ingramcontent.com/pod-product-compliance
Lightning Source LLC
Chambersburg PA
CBHW051447170526
45166CB00001B/152